Bio-Psycho-Social Contributions to Understanding Eating Disorders

Yael Latzer · Daniel Stein
Editors

Bio-Psycho-Social Contributions to Understanding Eating Disorders

Springer

Editors
Yael Latzer
Faculty of Social Welfare and Health Sciences
Haifa University
Mount Carmel Haifa
Israel

Daniel Stein
Faculty of Medicine
Tel Aviv University
Tel Aviv-Yafo
Israel

ISBN 978-3-319-32740-2 ISBN 978-3-319-32742-6 (eBook)
DOI 10.1007/978-3-319-32742-6

Library of Congress Control Number: 2016941085

Printed on acid-free paper

This Springer imprint is published by Springer Nature
The registered company is Springer International Publishing AG Switzerland

Contents

About the Editors

Yael Latzer, DSc, graduated from the University of Haifa with both her BA and MA degrees in Clinical Social Work. This was followed by obtaining her Doctor of Science (DSc) at the Technion Medical School in Haifa, Israel. She received additional certification in psychotherapy, family and couple therapy. She held a two-year (1989–1991) fellowship position, training in the treatment of eating disorders at the Psychoanalytic Institute, Menninger Foundation, in Topeka, Kansas, USA.

She founded the Institute for the Treatment and Study of Eating Disorders in the Division of Psychiatry at Rambam Health Care Campus, Haifa, Israel in 1992 and has since served as its director. She is currently Full Professor in the Faculty of Social Welfare and Health Sciences at the University of Haifa. Professor Latzer has served as the head of various academic programs, including a family therapy MA program, a clinical program, and most recently, MA program for oultra orthodox. She also developed an MA nutrition program, which was opened in 2008 with an emphasis on behavioral and psychological related factors, and has been the head of the program for 5 years.

Professor Latzer has published more than a 150 articles in scientific and clinical journals, as well as more than 50 chapters in various books. She has edited three books on varied topics of EDs. She has actively participated in many international and national scientific conferences and serves as a reviewer for a variety of international and local scientific journals. She was also nominated and served as the president of the Israeli Academy of Eating Disorders for 5 years. Her main topics of interest include sleeping and EDs, EDs and family, EDs and religiosity and EDs and identifying at-risk groups and prevention of EDs among Israeli adolescents subgroups prevention. She specializes in family-based treatment, cognitive behavioral therapy, and Interpersonal psychotherapy for EDs.

Five years ago Prof. Latzer developed and established an innovative project in Israel, the rehabilitation house for young women with eating disorders who have entered their recovery phase of treatment. ("Zeida Laderech"). In addition, over the last 10 years she have been active as an advisor to the Israeli Parliament ("Knesset") taking part in many meetings, and has contributed dramatically to the change in treatment policy regarding eating disorders. From 2010 to 2012 she served as advisor to pass a new Bill through the Israeli parliament, prohibiting the appearance of underweight models in commercial advertising.

Professor Latzer is both nationally and internationally recognized as an expert in the field of eating disorder treatment and research.

E-mail: latzery@gmail.com
Website: http://hw.haifa.ac.il/social/cv/Yael_Latzer.html
Professor, Faculty of Social Welfare and Health Sciences, Haifa University, Israel.
Director, Eating Disorders Institute, Psychiatric Division, Rambam Medical Center, Haifa, Israel.
Work: +972-(0)4-7773143
Cell: +972-(0)54-4736673
Cell USA: 1-917-9351824

Daniel Stein, MD, is a certified psychiatrist and child and adolescent psychiatrist. Since 1998, he is Director of the Pediatric Psychosomatic Department, Edmond and Lily Safra Children's Hospital, Chaim Sheba Medical Center, Tel Hashomer, Israel. He is Full Professor (clinical) at the Department of Psychiatry, and Head of the Section of Child and Adolescent Psychiatry at the Sackler Faculty of Medicine, University of Tel Aviv, Tel Aviv, Israel. His main topics of interest include child and adolescent psychiatry, eating disorders, psychosomatic and somatopsychic disorders, and suicidology. He specializes in psychodynamic psychotherapy and cognitive behavioral therapy. Professor Stein is a member of numerous Israeli and international organizations, including the International Society of Child and Adolescent Psychiatry, the Academy of Eating Disorders, the Eating Disorders Research Society, and the European College of Neuropsychiatry. He has participated in numerous international conferences and won several scientific awards. He is the co-founder and previous deputy chairman of the Israeli Academy of Eating Disorders and a reviewer in several important Israeli and international peer-reviewed journals. He has written more than 150 articles and book chapters published in prominent international journals and books, and is the co-editor of three books on the field of eating disorders. Dr. Stein is locally and internationally recognized as an expert in the field of eating disorder treatment and research.

Prof. Daniel Stein, MD,
Psychiatrist and Child and Adolescent Psychiatrist
Director, Pediatric Psychosomatic Department
Edmond and Lily Safra Children's Hospital
Chaim Sheba Medical Center, Tel Hashomer
Sackler Faculty of Medicine, Tel Aviv University, Tel Aviv, Israel
Tel: 972-03-5302690
Cell: 972-052-6666330
E-mail: prof.daniel.stein@gmail.com
Website: www.safra.sheba.co.il/pediatric psychosomatic department

About the Faculty of Social Welfare Health Science

The Faculty of Social Welfare and Health Sciences was established in 1996 by the University of Haifa and the Council for Higher Education. The impetus for its founding was the intense and rapid professionalization in Israel and throughout the world of the various disciplines encompassed by the faculty. In addition, the new faculty reflects the need for an academic institution of higher learning in the north of Israel to train professionals in the areas of social welfare and health sciences.

Following its establishment, the Faculty of Social Welfare and Health Sciences has strengthened cooperation and collaboration between the University of Haifa and the Technion and the Rappaport Faculty of Medicine by offering specialization in the areas of behavioral sciences and administration, on the one hand, and medical sciences on the other. Each institution contributes and gains from the programs.

At present, the Faculty of Social Welfare and Health Sciences includes the School of Social Work, the School of Public Health, the Department of Human Services, the Department of Occupational Therapy, the Department of Nursing, the Department of Physical Therapy, and the Department of Gerontology.

The Institute for the Treatment and Study of Eating Disorders was founded in 1992 as part of the Division of Psychiatry at Rambam Health Care Campus in Haifa, Israel. Professor Yael Latzer, who founded the eating disorders Institute, has been the director since its establishment. The center serves as a nationwide referral center (though its clients are primarily from the north of Israel), specializing in the assessment, diagnosis, and treatment of eating disorders in adolescents and adults. An average of 12 new patients is referred every week, and approximately 130 new patients are treated yearly. The clinic treatment model is based on a multidisciplinary framework with a focus on family-based treatment and cognitive behavior therapy. Based on this model, the clinic provides a two-year continuing education program for experienced clinicians from all disciplines. The institute has undergone an enormous amount of professional and clinical development over the years and has become a recognized leader in the field of eating disorders, both within Israel and in the international professional community.

The eating disorders Institute is affiliated with the Faculty of Social Welfare and Health Sciences at the University of Haifa, providing a training, practicum, and research setting for BA, MA, and PhD students. As a university-affiliated teaching department, the clinic trains students from different professions and conducts research projects on many diverse topics related to eating disorders.

Recently, the Institute launched a rehabilitation program for young women with eating disorders who have entered their recovery phase of treatment. This pioneering and unique program, supported by the National Insurance Institute of Israel and approved by the Ministry of Health and Ministry of Social Affairs and Social Services, aims to provide residence in a hostel setting for eating disorder patients during their recovery period. The house, "Zeyda Laderech," was opened in July 2009.

Yael Latzer, DSc, Eating Disorders Clinic Rambam Medical Center, Haifa, Israel University of Haifa, Faculty of Social Welfare and Health Sciences, Mount Carmel, Haifa, 31905 Israel. E-mail: latzer@zahav.net.il

Correspondence:
Prof. Yael Latzer DSc.
Professor, Faculty of Social Welfare and Health Sciences, Haifa University, Mount Carmel, Haifa, 31905 Israel.
Director, Eating Disorders Clinic, Psychiatric Division, Rambam Medical Center, Haifa, Israel.
E-mail: latzery@gmail.com
Work: +972-777-3143
Cell: +972-(0)54-4736673
Cell UAS: 1-917-935-1824

About the Pediatric Psychosomatic Department

The Pediatric Psychosomatic Department at the Edmond and Lily Safra Children's Hospital, Chaim Sheba Medical Center, Tel Hashomer, Israel, was founded in 1987 by Edith Mitrani MD. Serving as a nationwide referral center, this department specializes in the treatment of eating disorders in children and adolescents. Twenty patients are hospitalized at each period of time and around 80 patients are hospitalized yearly. The department runs a halfway-out day center and an ambulatory follow-up service. The halfway-out day center serves between 15–20 patients at each period of time and between 40–50 patients are treated there every year. The ambulatory clinic currently treats around 250 patients yearly. The department has treated over 1300 patients since its foundation.

Treatment is based on behavioral rehabilitation of disordered eating performed by a multi-professional team. Patients receive specialized individual, family, and group therapies. Treatment is geared toward the amelioration of disordered eating preoccupations and behaviors, alongside treating comorbid disturbances and promoting the ongoing developmental needs of the adolescent. Treatment is also geared toward encouraging appropriate changes in the family to consolidate the changes achieved and to reduce the risk for relapse.

As a university-affiliated teaching department, the Pediatric Psychosomatic Department trains students from different professions. The department runs many research projects in diverse topics related to eating disorders, suicidality, and psychosocial aspects of pediatric medical disorders.

Correspondence:
Prof. Daniel Stein, MD
Director, Pediatric Psychosomatic Department
Edmond and Lily Safra Children's Hospital
Chaim Sheba Medical Center, IL-5265601 Tel Hashomer, Israel
E-mails: prof.daniel.stein@gmail.com; daniel,stein@sheba.health.gov.il
Phone: +972-(0) 3-5302690; Cell: +972-(0) 52-6666330
Website: www.safra.sheba.co.il/pediatric psychosomatic department

Introduction

Eating disorders (EDs) are considered a major problem of the modern era, ranking among the most prevailing public health issues facing female adolescents and young adults in many countries around the globe [1]. Despite the abundance of research investigating many aspects relevant to EDs in the last two decades, ED patients, their families, their treatment providers, and the society in which they live continue to experience a multitude of problems. These include detrimental myths and prejudices as well as the interference of political considerations with respect to the budgets provided for treatment, research, and prevention.

These issues are of particular relevance in Israel because, on the one hand, since the 1990s, Israeli male and female youngsters have been troubled with eating-related disturbances to a greater extent than many other Western industrialized countries [2], raising critical questions about their emotional well-being. Yet, on the other hand, the funding provided for the treatment of EDs in Israel is scarce relative to almost all other Western industrialized countries [3]. This gap between needs and resources led us to invite key distinguished researchers from around the globe to collaborate with local Israeli researchers in the vital endeavor of systematically tackling major unanswered issues in the ED field via a comprehensive book series. We previously edited two books resulting from this multinational endeavor, with implications for ED stakeholders around the world. The first book deals with historical and sociocultural aspects of EDs, and it also spans vast multidimensional and interdisciplinary literature with respect to different etiological theories for EDs. The second book summarizes a similarly comprehensive endeavor with respect to treatment for and outcome of EDs [4, 5].

The current book is geared toward specific issues related to EDs that are relatively new to the field, yet in our opinion hold considerable importance. In this book, we aimed to integrate three different aspects of these novel contributions: medical, psychological, and sociocultural. It is our hope that readers of our book will gain a more holistic perspective not only on the role of each facet but also on their interplay in order to promote the understanding, treatment, prevention, and research of EDs.

Medical Aspects of Eating Disorders

In this era, EDs are conceptualized as partly representing genetically transmitted disorders [6] associated with a variety of altered brain functions [7]. The first two chapters in this book that discuss the association of EDs with attention deficit hyperactivity disorder (ADHD) and with sleeping disorders, respectively, point toward this conceptualization. The next two chapters discuss medical issues that result from EDs: osteoporosis and skeletal involvement in general.

Chapter 1 *Attention Deficit Hyperactivity Disorder (ADHD) and Eating Disorders* (Kaplan et al.)

Allan Kaplan and his associates from the University of Toronto in Canada are among the most prominent researchers studying the relations between EDs and ADHD. Until recently, the links between the two entities were relatively neglected. To correct this flaw, Kaplan et al.'s chapter reviews the growing body of research that has begun to examine the overlap in neurocognitive dysfunction, epidemiology, and genetics that characterize both EDs and ADHD. First and foremost, evidence indicates elevated rates of childhood ADHD in individuals who later develop EDs, particularly but not only for the bingeing/purging spectrum [8]. Moreover, overweight children show a greater preponderance of ADHD inattention symptoms, for example deficits in set shifting, as well as of impulsivity, in comparison to normal-weight youngsters [9]. Kaplan et al. highlight the abundant ADHD-related cognitive disturbances found in youngsters with EDs, including disturbances in executive functions such as impulse control, organizational and attentional capabilities, cognitive flexibility, set shifting, problem solving, decision making, and working memory [10, 11]. These disturbances are related to physiological dysfunction of the medial prefrontal cortex, orbitofrontal cortex, anterior cingulate cortex, and striatum [12, 13]. They may exert a deleterious effect on the integration of the process of eating; they may also increase the rigidity and obsessionality of weight- and shape-related cognitions [14] and the urges and impulsive behaviors associated with binge eating. Some of these disturbances may persist even in ED patients achieving long-term weight restoration and normal eating behaviors [11, 13], suggesting that they may be core ED traits that are independent of the effect of malnutrition and erratic eating patterns. Moreover, Kaplan et al.'s chapter summarizes molecular genetic studies, proposing that common genes involved in dopamine transport are found in binge eating, obesity, and ADHD, likely suggesting a shared genetic predisposition. These findings suggest that methylphenidate, which potentially improves ADHD-related cognitive disturbances, may have some beneficial effect on ED-related cognitions and behaviors. Although evidence-based support for this contention is not yet available, a few case reports administering methylphenidate to ED patients (mainly bulimia nervosa—BN) have shown promising results (e.g., [15]).

Chapter 2 *Sleeping Disorders in Eating Disorder Patients* (Latzer and Tzicshinsky)

The third chapter in this book, written by Yael Latzer from the Haifa University, and from Rambam Medical center in Israel and Orna Tzicshinsky from the Emek Yezreel Academic College in Israel, deals with another important neurologically related issue: the relationship between disturbances in eating and sleeping among adolescents. Eating and sleeping are both basic needs of the human body that are essential for normal development and existence. These needs are directly connected and mutually influence one another. Every situation that involves a physiological and mental imbalance may manifest itself in eating and sleeping patterns, especially when transitioning from one life stage to another. The intensity and the nature of the reaction may differ from one person to another and may be affected by the individual's genetic predisposition, personality, length and magnitude of the change, and social and cultural environment. The first part of this chapter describes both normative and pathological eating and sleeping development and behavior. In the second part, the authors discuss studies examining sleep–wake patterns among adolescents suffering from EDs. Finally, the importance of maintaining a balance between adolescents' needs for autonomy and the supervision and support of parents as providers of healthy nutrition and sleeping habits is discussed.

Chapters 3 and 4 *Osteoporosis and Skeletal Involvement in Eating Disorders* (Zuckerman et al.)

Nehama Zuckerman et al. from the Rambam Medical center in Haifa, Israel, discuss in Chap. 5 the hormonal derangements involved in the physiological disturbances characterizing the ED spectrum, ranging from malnourishment to morbid obesity. The hormonal disturbances in EDs involve the growth hormone–insulin-like growth factor (GH–IGF) axis, with its influence on growth and bone metabolism, which are of particular relevance in adolescents. Involvement of the hypothalamic-pituitary-gonadal axis is common in girls and boys with EDs, demonstrating delayed puberty or hypogonadotrophic hypogonadism and amenorrhea. Hypercortisolemia, abnormal hypothalamic-pituitary-thyroid axis, and osmoregulation alterations also occur.

In Chap. 4, the authors focus on a main concern regarding the endocrinological instability of patients with EDs: the effect of malnourishment and abnormal eating on the skeleton, in particular the risk of decreased bone mineral density (BMD). EDs place adolescents and young adults at risk for bone loss or failure to attain appropriate peak bone mass. Zuckerman and her colleagues emphasize that even in individuals who have suffered from an ED during adolescence and are not symptomatic as adults, not to mention patients with chronic EDs, there is still an increased risk of bone pain and fractures. Adolescents suffering from EDs may evince, in addition, an increased risk of stress fractures and kyphoscoliosis, and many do not achieve their expected final height [16]. This chapter further highlights that one of the reasons for the reduced BMD in anorexia nervosa (AN) patients, in addition to reduced mineral intake and amenorrhea, is their low bone turnover, with relatively higher osteoclastic (bone resorptive) than osteoblasic (bone formation) activity. By contrast, normal-weight BN is not associated with low BMD, unless there is a past history of AN.

Zuckerman and her associates conduct an extensive review of the literature, while adding their own clinical and research input to the continuous discussion of whether to add hormones to the treatment of patients with AN to reduce the risk of osteoporosis. They firmly emphasize that treatment modalities involving hormonal supplements have limited effectiveness, whereas increased caloric intake and resumption of menses are essential to improved BMD. Lastly, bone loss may not be completely reversible in recovered AN patients. This accentuates the great importance of early diagnosis for the establishment of appropriate target weight range (based on premorbid rather than on current weight and height), and for vigorous weight restoration during adolescence [16].

Psychological Aspects of Eating Disorders

Next, three chapters in this book introduce psychological aspects of EDs, followed by two chapters examining specific psychological treatment interventions in EDs. The study of psychological factors potentially predisposing an individual to an ED is subject to considerable conceptual and methodological controversies and ambiguities. Different psychological models relate differently to the etiology of EDs, as in the case of any psychopathology of a putative psycho-developmental origin, according to specific built-in conceptualizations that are generated from treatments of already-ill individuals. The inherent problems with such models in the case of an ED are, first, that hypotheses about predisposing psychological factors are derived from findings in patients who are severely ill not only psychologically but also physiologically when analyzed, and, second, that these models cannot be subjected to rigorous research. Despite these limitations, the merit of any psychological model is that it may assist at least some ED patients (and their therapists) in understanding that their suffering has some relevant deep-rooted personal meaning; this, in turn, may offer an opportunity towards self-acceptance, and/or readiness for change. The current book contains chapters focusing on psychological experiences that are of considerable relevance in ED patients—suicide (Chap. 5), trans-generational transmission of disordered emotional difficulties (Chap. 6), and pathological altruism (Chap. 8).

Chapter 5 *Suicide in Eating Disorders* (Lilenfeld)

In this chapter, Lisa Lilenfeld from the Argosy University, Washington D.C., USA critically reviews the literature on suicide and attempted suicide in EDs. She emphasizes that the mortality rate among ED patients has substantially increased in comparison to healthy control populations, in particular among patients with AN, with standardized mortality ratios ranging from 2.9 to 17.8 [17, 18]. Suicide in AN usually appears within 10 years after the onset of the illness. Suicide is the second leading cause of death in AN patients, after the complications of the ED itself [19]. The picture is less consistent in the case of BN. Whereas in several studies suicide appears to represent the most frequent cause of death in BN, above and beyond the medical complications of the disorder [20]; some prospective outcome studies have not found elevated suicide rates in patients diagnosed with BN in comparison to healthy controls [21], a position also held by Lilenfeld in this chapter.

With respect to attempted suicide, current research suggests that the frequency of attempted suicide and the medical severity of suicide attempts in AN and BN [22] are comparable to those found in major depression and conduct disorder, and are greater than those found in schizophrenia and anxiety disorders. However, in contrast to the findings for completed suicide, suicide attempts and parasuicidal behaviors are more prevalent and pose a greater problem in BN and binge/purge type AN (AN-B/P) than in restrictive AN (AN-R) patients [19].

Lilenfeld summarizes that several factors have been repeatedly shown to increase suicidal risk in EDs. These include the severity of the ED symptomatology, the presence of binge/purge symptomatology, comorbid depression, anxiety, substance use disorders, and personality disorders (particularly, although not only, borderline personality disorder), elevated impulsivity, severe body image and perception disturbances, a history of sexual abuse, and past suicide attempts [19, 22, 23]. Some suggest that whereas depression may be associated with elevated suicidal risk in AN-R adolescents, elevated impulsivity, violence, and aggression may characterize suicidal behavior in individuals with impulse control disturbances, including BN and AN-B/P [24].

Lilenfeld underscores the importance of in-depth suicide assessment for every ED patient, to include the suicide risk factors described above as well as relevant protective factors such as the likelihood of familial and social support. Such an assessment should be an integral part not only of the initial evaluation of the ED patient but also during the ongoing process of treatment. With respect to treatment, Lilenfeld emphasizes that in addition to managing the causes leading to suicide attempt and dealing with familial and social antecedents, two important processes must be taken into consideration: what the patient expects to achieve when attempting suicide, and the development of alternative skills and coping strategies to better deal with the problems leading to the suicidal act.

Chapter 6 *Mothers with eating disorders: The environmental factors affecting eating-related emotional difficulties in their offspring* (Sadeh-Sarvit et al.)

In this chapter, Shiry Sade-Sharvit and her colleagues from the Bar Ilan and Haifa Universities, the Shalvata and Sheba Medical Centers and the Interdisciplinary Center in Israel study the way in which mothers suffering from EDs function with their toddlers, particularly with respect to the toddlers' eating patterns. The study, based on an object-relations psychodynamic perspective, uses semi-structured interviews conducted with the mothers. It shows that early needs of mothers with EDs that were unmet by their own parents, alongside exaggerated anxiety about their children's eating and weight, are experienced mostly in mothers' relationships with their daughters, but not with their sons. This may, in turn, increase the risk of inadequate maternal feeding practices, and of maternal anxieties about the daughter becoming overweight. These findings imply that female children of mothers with EDs are at greater risk of becoming a second generation experiencing eating- and weight-related emotional difficulties. Needless to say, the findings of this research study are only preliminary and speculative. Prospective longitudinal research, including both mothers with EDs and a control group without EDs, should be undertaken to enable a more in-depth understanding of the role of maternal ED in the offspring's predisposition toward maladaptive eating- and weight-related attitudes and behaviors.

Chapter 7 *Eating Disorders and Pathological Altruism* (Bachner-Melman and Oakley)

Rachel Bachner-Melman from the Rupin Academic Center in Israel and Barbara Oakley from the Oakland University in Rochester, Missouri, USA discuss whether individuals suffering from an ED can be conceptualized as representing prototypical pathological altruism. The theoretical concept of "pathological altruism" in patients with an ED has its roots in self-psychology paradigms [25, 26]. Accordingly, in an attempt to enhance a vulnerable sense of self-worth, the future patient with an ED is geared toward renunciation of his/her own needs, i.e., to act as a selfless individual [25, 26], in order to serve the needs of significant others. In this chapter, Bachner-Melman and Oakley extend their conceptualization from giving up one's own needs (selflessness) to sacrificing one's whole sense of self at the service of others (pathological altruism). This paradigm is based on the understanding that both genetic and environmental factors may contribute to a poorly defined sense of self and the resulting adaptation to external expectations and devotion to others' needs. When the willingness to place another's perceived needs above one's own occurs in a way that may cause self-harm, the normally nurturing, positive, and necessary characteristic of altruism can become pathological. The authors further elaborate that the endorsement of the thin beauty ideal underlying the predisposition to an ED may be conceptualized as a form of pathological altruism because the biological need to eat is sacrificed to fulfill the "needs" or dictates of the society at large concerning this body ideal. The authors provide theoretical, clinical, and empirical data that lends support to their paradigm, and they offer relevant suggestions with respect to outcome, treatment, and prevention.

Psychological Treatment in Eating Disorders

From a treatment-related perspective, structured time-limited manualized treatment models, such as cognitive behavioral therapy (CBT) [27] and dialectic behavioral therapy (DBT) [28], have gained considerable acceptance in the treatment of EDs, particularly in patients diagnosed with binge/purge symptoms. These relatively short-term here-and-now symptom-oriented interventions seem to appeal to ED patients, who are often not psychologically oriented. Moreover, these strategies can be subjected to randomized controlled trials in comparison to other relevant treatments or to a waitlisted condition. Nonetheless, one psychodynamics-related therapy, self-psychology, is considered appealing to the ED patient because it aims to enhance a very important personal dimension—self-esteem, and it has been investigated in controlled randomized research [25].

Nonetheless, several perspectives should be taken into consideration when it comes to the treatment of EDs. In keeping with the biological shared vulnerability of different ED subtypes [29], these subtypes also share significant psychological traits [30]. Moreover, several core ED-related dimensions are at the heart of different psychological treatment models. These include severe personality-related pathology (see Bruch [31]) and neurocognitive disturbances [11] which are likely involved in all treatment modalities, as well as disturbances in self-esteem (self-psychology and CBT), affect and impulse regulation (CBT and DBT), and social relationships/capacities (CBT and self-psychology). Lastly, with the exception of family-based therapy in younger patients with a relatively short duration of illness [32], there is no evidence for the superiority of one treatment intervention over another in AN, with most therapies showing modest effect at best [33]. Moreover, while CBT is by far the most empirically supported treatment strategy in EDs, the picture is quite different when it comes to clinical practice. Thus, psychotherapists have been found to use mostly a non-structured and somewhat vague combination of both psychodynamic and cognitive behavioral principles, which are often quite diverse among different therapists [34]. The present book includes two chapters that critically analyze specialized, relatively unique treatment interventions for ED patients: an integrative treatment approach for ED women with a history sexual abuse (Chap. 8) and a skill sharing intervention for families (Chap. 9).

Chapter 8 *An Integrative Treatment Approach in Women with an Eating Disorder and a History of Sexual Abuse* (Zubery et al.)

In this chapter, Eynat Zubery from the Shalvata Medical Center in Israel, Yael Latzer from the Haifa University and from Rambam Medical Center in Israel, and Daniel Stein from the Sheba Medical Center and Tel Aviv University in Israel propose a practice-based model for the treatment of patients suffering from EDs in the context of a history of childhood sexual abuse (CSA). It is now recognized that many women suffering from an ED have experienced some form of sexual abuse during their childhood. It is of note that a history of CSA is more prevalent in patients with EDs diagnosed with binge/purge behaviors than in restricting type EDs [35]. Moreover, binge/purge behaviors may be conceptualized as a means to alleviate the pain associated with the traumatic event similar to self-injurious behaviors or to substance abuse. Accordingly, the treatment of patients with coexisting ED and CSA showing binge/purge pathology may proceed along different lines than the treatment of patients with restrictive-type EDs and a history of CSA.

Our model includes three stages. Differences in the treatment of binge/purge and restrictive patients with EDs and CSA are found primarily in the first stage dealing mainly with ED-related and other symptomatic disturbances. Supportive therapy or psychodynamic therapy is recommended in patients with restrictive-type EDs along with dietetic counseling, whereas CBT and/or DBT are recommended for binge/purge type EDs. It is assumed that stabilization of ED-related and other comorbid symptoms has to be achieved before trauma-related issues can be effectively worked through.

The second phase, relating mainly to the CSA and its past, present, and future implications, involves individual psychodynamic therapy for the patients, separate psychodynamic group counseling for parents, and family therapy for the whole family, in cases where family members do not represent a threat to the patient. The separate treatment modules create a therapeutic space for both the patient and family for the disclosure of the CSA. The fundamentals of this stage relate to the need to empower the patients by decreasing their social isolation and sense of helplessness and by increasing the range of adaptive options offered for effective handling of trauma-related issues [36]. It is also based on the premise that disturbances associated with post-traumatic stress disorder (PTSD) resulting from a single trauma are highly different from complex PTSD resulting from prolonged interpersonal abuse such as CSA [36].

In the third phase, patients continue working through trauma-elicited material carried out in individual and/or group formats. To summarize, the authors suggest that an integrative approach dealing at the start with ED-related and other comorbid symptoms and thereafter with trauma-related issues may have sound theoretical and clinical implications in the treatment of patients with coexisting ED and a history of CSA [37].

Chapter 9 *Interpersonal Maintaining Factors in Eating Disorders: Skill Sharing Interventions for Carers* (Treasure et al.)

Janet Treasure and her associates from King's College, Institute of Psychiatry and South London and Maudsley NHS Trust, London, United Kingdom describe an intervention designed to share information and skills with carers of people with an ED. At the start, the authors summarize the evidence that family support and lack of familial criticism toward patients with EDs may contribute to good outcomes, whereas disturbed family relationships increase the risk for poor outcome. The authors then propose a model, based on extensive research data, to explain these findings (see 38). According to this model, the liability of relatives to share with the patient personal vulnerability dispositions such as obsessionlity, rigidity, elevated anxiety, and avoidance—alongside the propensity of a prolonged waning and waxing illness such as an ED to induce negative feelings of criticism, hostility, overprotection (i.e., elevated expressed emotion, see Kyriacou et al. [39]), frustration, shame, and guilt among family members—may combine to reduce the likelihood for change, likely maintaining the ED for a prolonged period.

In the second part of the chapter, the authors emphasize that the likelihood of family members to either reinforce and maintain an ED, or conversely, to increase the likelihood of recovery, necessitates the development of interventions in which relatives act as recovery-supporting coaches. This is based on the premise that although carers may lack information and skills, they are still highly motivated to contribute to the recovery of their relative with an ED. Treasure and her associates have developed a short-term manual-based treatment program for this purpose. In this intervention, facilitators provide information and teach skills that aim to improve the carers' adaptive coping (e.g., assisting their ill relative in taking the appropriate care over her eating) as well as training carers to reduce potentially illness-maintaining behaviors (e.g., to avoid cooperating with the hiding of binge/purge behaviors). The process of family training in this program includes theoretical considerations such as sharing information about health behavior change processes, a functional analysis of personal and familial ED-maintaining behaviors, and the teaching of skills such as refined communication. Thus, the carers are taught skills to change their own behaviors and attitudes toward their relative with an ED, as well as to teach these skills to the patient and thereby assist her to achieve her own desired improvement.

In the last part of the chapter, the authors provide information from an open pilot study and a randomized study of this skills-sharing manual versus another form of family intervention. They conclude that this intervention is acceptable to the carers, and that its content and structure are judged as relevant and useful. Moreover, the treatment was found to reduce the carers' distress and caregiving difficulties. However, no data is available yet about the influence of the intervention on the condition of the patients.

Social Aspects of Eating Disorder

Traditionally, EDs have been conceptualized to represent a culture-dependent syndrome, namely a syndrome that cannot be understood separately from its cultural context, and that is restricted to a limited number of cultures by virtue of specific psychosocial factors [40]. Studies supporting this view flourished between the 1960s and the 1980s. More recent research, however, casts doubt as to the definition of EDs as culturally dependent [41] because, for example, of the relative infrequency of full-blown EDs in comparison to the high frequency of females' dissatisfaction with their weight and preoccupation with dieting [29]. Still, some suggest that rather than completely disregarding the wealth of literature associating EDs with culture, these disorders might be conceptualized as a cultural byproduct of modernity that has a role in genetically, biologically, and psychologically predisposed individuals [42]. EDs are attributed in this context to a combination of socioeconomic developments, including the rapidly changing roles of women and the considerable distress associated with this change; the sociocultural emphasis on thinness that currently cuts across many cultures; and the shift in eating patterns resulting from the recent advent of modernity and changes in food availability in many regions across the globe [42].

In line with this conceptualization, the last four chapters of this book relate to sociocultural aspects associated with EDs. The first chapter in this section deals with the provision of emotional first-aid to people suffering from EDs. The second chapter deals with the growing influence of pro-anorexia (pro-ana) websites in recent years on eating-, weight-, and shape-related attitudes and behaviors of young people. The last two chapters deal with religious aspects related to EDs. One chapter associates historical background with modern conceptualizations in discussing the issue of "spiritual self-starvation" or "holy anorexia" in the context of the "Jerusalem Syndrome." The second chapter deals with the protective role of religious orientation and spirituality in reducing the risk for the development and maintenance of disordered eating in young individuals. To summarize, we suggest that with the flourishing of neurogenetic models with regard to the predisposition and maintenance of EDs, social processes may still have an important role in the understanding of the changes envisioned in the presentation, prognosis, and treatment of EDs in the past decades.

Chapter 10 *Emotional First-Aid in Eating Disorders: The Unique Role of Hotlines and Online Services* (Gilat and Latzer)

Itzhak Gilat from the Levinsky Academic College in Israel and Yael Latzer from the Haifa University and Rambam Medical Center in Israel note that over the past decades, volunteer-based hotlines and online services have become an attractive source for emotional first-aid around the globe. These services may specifically play an important role for individuals with EDs, as they require less psychological involvement from the client than professional interventions. This is of particular relevance both for AN patients, who are often reluctant to share their emotions and distress with professionals [43], and for BN patients who often feel ashamed and disgusted by their illness [44]. The therapeutic potential of hotline and online services for patients with EDs is demonstrated in this chapter by means of empirical analyses of the experiences brought forward by the users. The authors conclude that hotline and online services may pave the way for the reluctant patient with an ED toward later professional therapy, and may offer additional support for patients who are already under treatment.

Chapter 11 *The Characteristics of Pro-Ana Communities* (Boniel-Nissim and Latzer)

In this chapter, Meyran Boniel-Nissim and Yael Latzer from Haifa University in Israel aim to identify the characteristics of pro-ana communities and to understand the motivations underlining individuals' engagement in these websites. In particular, the authors emphasize the influence of pro-ana communities in the development and maintenance of an ED via the mechanism of the "contagious" social learning experience. The authors further suggest that the need of adolescents to identify with role models and to belong to their own subculture in the process of the second separation and individuation process [45] becomes of particular relevance in youngsters suffering from an ED, who are often socially isolated and highly desperate and self-critical. In this respect, pro-ana communities presented on websites are designed to encourage these youngsters to regard their ED as representing their self-identity and chosen lifestyle rather than as a disease, and to shun the influence of treatment, treatment providers, and the outside world in general [46]. Common features of these websites include support groups, forums and chat rooms, tips and tricks (to lose weight and to conceal disordered eating from others), the use of specific secretive jargon, e.g., "thinspiration" and "reverse thinspiration" images, as well as the provision of links to other similar pro-ana websites. One of the most common and disconcerting aspects of these websites is the detailed instructions for initiating and maintaining the ED. Pro-ana members join a special target-based virtual community that does not denounce weight loss and self-starvation but rather encourages and strengthens disordered ED-related cognitions and behaviors. Moreover, under certain conditions, pro-ana groups may reach the proportion of a secretive cult.

Chapter 12 *Spiritual Self Starvation En-Route to Salvation* (Witztum et al.)

In this chapter Eliezer Witztum from the Mental Health Center, Beer Sheva, Division of Psychiatry, and the Faculty of Health Sciences, Ben-Gurion University of the Negev, Beer Sheva, in Israel, Daniel Stein from the Sheba Medical Center and Tel Aviv University, Israel, Yael Latzer from the Haifa University and Rambam Medical Center in Israel, and Mohse Kalian, the former District Psychiatrist in Jerusalem, Israel, discuss at the start the historical background of the relationships between disordered eating and religious and symbolic idioms. Subsequently, the phenomenon termed "spiritual self-starvation" and its linkage to asceticism is described in the context of religious beliefs and practices. The religious aspects of this phenomenon are further elaborated via three cases demonstrating the appearance of highly disordered eating-related attitudes and behaviors in people diagnosed with the so-called "Jerusalem Syndrome." Accordingly, their extraordinary visit to Jerusalem has led these individuals to induced fasting and voluntary refusal to eat in the context of sacredness, purification, and penance. The afflicted individuals perceive their distress in terms that construct a narrative integrating self-starvation into their religious and spiritual life. "Spiritual self-starvation" in these cases exceeds the boundaries of religious devoutness to the extent of self-endangering psychotic attitudes and behaviors. The authors conclude that the significance of Jerusalem as a unique sacred space where, according to religious eschatology, great events are about to occur, may lead premorbidly vulnerable individuals to enactments that are reflected in their utilization of the holy space for personal salvation as well as for global redemption.

Chapter 13 *The Influence of Religious Orientation and Spiritual Well-Being on Body Dissatisfaction and Disordered Eating in a Sample of Jewish Women* (Weinberger-Litman et al.)

Complex interactions may exist between religion and health-related problems [47], including those related to self-starvation and disordered eating [48]. In this chapter, Sarah Weinberger-Litman and her associates from the Brooklyn College, the Graduate Center of the City University of New York, and the Mount Sinai School of Medicine, New York, NY and the Reading Hospital and Medical Center, Reading, PA, in the USA suggest that in modern religious practice, a greater level of religiosity may protect the individual from disordered eating. In particular, women characterized as intrinsically religious, namely who incorporate the role of religion as guiding important aspects of their life [49], have been found to have less ED pathology in comparison to extrinsically religious women, in whom security and solace are the result of belonging to a specific religious community [50]. In support of this contention, Weinberger-Litman et al. have shown that in Jewish female adolescents and young women in New York, participants with an intrinsic religious orientation have less pathology on measures of body dissatisfaction and eating disturbances than women with an extrinsic religious orientation. Furthermore, the authors found that high levels of spiritual well-being contribute above and beyond the effect of religion per se to reduce body dissatisfaction but not disordered eating. These findings led Weinberger and her colleagues to conclude that an intrinsic spiritual religious orientation may potentially serve to protect women from body image disturbances.

Conclusions

In the present book, we have attempted to create a multifaceted, intriguing, yet balanced viewpoint in a field that develops and changes very rapidly. With the aim of broadening the knowledge and understanding of EDs and their management, we have included specific contributions on biological/medical, psychological, and sociocultural aspects of EDs that have been previously addressed only infrequently. Nevertheless, reading this book might leave us with more questions than answers. Ongoing discourses among clinicians and researchers specializing in diverse aspects related to EDs, like those gathered in this book, may allow for the continuation of fruitful, enterprising, and dialectic dialogues. We are fortunate that important international and Israeli researchers have agreed to contribute their innovative and state-of-the-art perspectives to this book, and we wish to extend our deep gratitude to all of them once again.

Yael Latzer
Daniel Stein

References

1. Hoek HW. Incidence, prevalence and mortality of anorexia nervosa and other eating disorders. Curr Opin Psychiatry. 2006;19:389–394.
2. Harel-Fisch Y, Walsh S, Djalovski A, Amit S, Tessler R, Haviv G. Health behaviors in school-aged children (HBSC) – a world health organization cross-national study. Israel: Bar-Ilan University, School of Education, 2011 (in Hebrew).
3. Latzer Y, Witztum E, Stein D. Eating disorders as an idiom of distress: The Israeli perspective. Eur J Eat Disord Rev. 2008;16:361–374.
4. Latzer Y, Merrick J, Stein D. editors. Understanding eating disorders: integrating culture, psychology and biology. New York: Nova Science Publishers Inc.; 2011.
5. Stein D, Latzer Y. editors. Treatment and Recovery of Eating Disorders. New York: Nova Science Publishers Inc.; 2012.
6. Klump KL, Miller KB, Keel PK, McGue M, Iacono WG. Genetic and environmental influences on anorexia nervosa syndromes in a population-based twin sample. Psychol Med 2001;31:737–740.
7. Kaye WH, Wagner A, Fudge JL, Paulus M. Neurocircuity of eating disorders. Curr Top Behav Neurosci. 2011;6:37–57
8. Biederman J, Ball SW, Monuteaux MC, Surman CB, Johnson JL, Zeitlin S. Are girls with ADHD at risk for eating disorders? Results from a controlled, five-year prospective study. J Dev Behav Pediatr. 2007;28:302–307.
9. Braet C, Claus L, Verbeken S, Van Vlierberghe, L. Impulsivity in overweight children. Eur Child Adolesc Psychiatry. 2007;16:473–483.

10. Green MW, Elliman NA, Wakeling A, Rogers PJ. Cognitive functioning, weight change and therapy in anorexia nervosa. J Psychiatr Res. 1996;30:401–410
11. Roberts ME, Tchanturia K, Stahl D, Southgate L, Treasure J. A systematic review and meta-analysis of set-shifting ability in eating disorders. Psyche Med. 2007;37:1075–1084
12. Uher R, Murphy T, Brammer MJ, Dalgleish T, Phillips ML, Ng VW, Andrew CM, Williams SC, Campbell IC. Treasure J. Medial prefrontal cortex activity associated with symptom provocation in eating disorders. Am J Psychiatry. 2004;161:1238–1246.
13. Oberndorfer TA, Kaye WH, Simmons AN, Strigo IA, Matthews SC. Demand-specific alteration of medial prefrontal cortex response during an inhibition task in recovered anorexic women. Int J Eat Disord. 2011;44:18.
14. Gillberg IC, Råstam M, Wentz E, Gillberg C. Cognitive and executive functions in anorexia nervosa ten years after onset of eating disorder. J Clin Exp Neuropsychol. 2007;29:170–178.
15. Drimmer EJ. Stimulant treatment of bulimia nervosa with and without attention-deficit disorder: three case reports. Nutrition. 2003;19:76–87.
16. Modan-Moses D, Yaroslavsky A, Novikov I, Segev S, Toledano A, Miterany E, Weizman A, Stein D. Stunting of growth as a major feature of anorexia nervosa in adolescent males. Pediatrics. 2003;111:270–276.
17. Keel PK, Dorer DJ, Eddy KT, Franko D, Charlatan DL, Herzog DB. Predictors of mortality in eating disorders. Arch Gen Psychiatry 2003;60:179–183.
18. Pompili M, Mancinelli I, Girardi P, Ruberto A, Tatarelli R. Suicide in anorexia nervosa: A meta-analysis. Int J Eat Disord. 2004;36:99–103.
19. Franko DL, Keel PK. Suicidality in eating disorders: Occurrence, correlates, and clinical implications. Clin Psychol Rev. 2006;26:769–782.
20. Mitchell JE, Pyle RL, Hatsukami D, Goff G, Glotter D, Harper J. A 2-5 year follow-up study of patients treated for bulimia. Int J Eat Disord. 1998;8:157–165.
21. Franko DL, Keel PK, Dorer DJ, Blais MA, Delinsky SS, Eddy KT, Charat V, Renn R, Herzog DB. What predicts suicide attempts in women with eating disorders? Psychol Med. 2004;34:843–853.
22. Mitchell JE, Pyle RL, Hatsukami D, Goff G, Glotter D, Harper J. A 2-5 year follow-up study of patients treated for bulimia. Int J Eat Disord. 1998;8:157–165.
23. Bulik CM, Thornton L, Pinheiro AP, Plotnicov KH, Klump KL, Brandt H, Crawford S, Fichter MM, Halmi KA, Johnson C, Kaplan AS, Mitchell J, Nutzinger D, Strober M, Treasure J, Woodside DB, Berrettini WH, Kaye WH.. Suicide attempts in anorexia nervosa. Psychosom Med. 2008;70:378–383.
24. Stein D, Lilenfeld LRR, Wildman PC, Marcus MD. Attempted suicide and self-injury in patients diagnosed with eating disorders. Compr Psychiatry. 2004;45:447–451.
25. Bachar E, Latzer Y, Kreitler S, Berry E. Empirical comparison of two psychological therapies: self psychology and cognitive orientation in the treatment of anorexia and bulimia. J Psychother Pract Res. 1999;8:115–128.
26. Apter A, Gothelf D, Orbach I, Weizman R, Ratzoni G, Har-Even D, Tyano S. Correlation of suicidal and violent behavior in different categories in hospitalized adolescent patients. J Am Acad Child Adolesc Psychiatry. 1995;34:912–918.
27. Agras WS, Walsh T, Fairburn CG, Wilson GT, Kramer HC. A multicenter comparison of cognitive-behavioral therapy and interpersonal psychotherapy for bulimia nervosa. Arch Gen Psychiatry. 2000;57:459–466.
30. Chen EY, Matthews L, Allen C, Kuo JR, Linehan MM. Dialectical behavior therapy for clients with binge-eating disorder or bulimia nervosa and borderline personality disorder. Int J Eat Disord. 2008;4:505–512.
31. Kaye W, Strober M, Jimerson D. The neurobiology of eating disorders. In: Charney DS, Nestler EJ, editors. The neurobiology of mental illness. New York: Oxford Press; 2004: 1112–1128.
32. Vitousek KM, Stumpf RE. Difficulties in the assessment of personality traits and disorders in eating-disordered individuals. Eat Disord. 2005;13:3760.

33. Bruch H. Eating disorders: Obesity, anorexia nervosa and the person within. New York: Basic Books; 1973.
34. Lock J, Le Grange D, Agras WS, Moye A, Bryson SW, Jo B. Randomized clinical trial comparing family-based treatment with adolescent-focused individual therapy for adolescents with anorexia nervosa. Arch Gen Psychiatry. 2010;67:1025–1032
35. Hartmann A, Weber S, Herpertz S, Zeeck A. Psychological treatment for anorexia nervosa: A meta-analysis of standardized mean change. Psychother Psychosom. 2011; 80:216–226.
36. Tobin, DL, Banker JB, Weisberg L, Bowers W. I know what you did last summer (and It was Not CBT): A factor analytic model of international psychotherapeutic practice in the eating disorders psychotherapeutic practice. Int J Eat Disord. 2007;40:754–767.
37. Goodsitt A: Eating disorders: A self-psychological perspective. In: Garner DM, Garfinkel PE, editors. Handbook of treatment for eating disorders. New York: Guilford Press; 1997:208–228
38. Wonderlich SA, Brewerton TD, Jocic Z, Dansky BS, Abbott DW. The relationship of childhood sexual abuse and eating disorders: A review. J Am Acad Child Adolesc Psychiatry. 1997;36:1107–1115.
39. Herman JL. Trauma and recovery. New York: Basic Books; 1992.
40. Brewerton TD. Eating disorders, trauma, and comorbidity: Focus on PTSD. Eat Disord. 2007;15:285–304.
41. Schmidt U, Treasure J. Anorexia nervosa: Valued and visible. A cognitive-interpersonal maintenance model and its implications for research and practice. Br J Clin Psychol. 2006;45:125.
42. Kyriacou O, Treasure J, Schmidt U. Expressed emotion in eating disorders assessed via self-report. An examination of factors associated with expressed emotion in careres of people with anorexia nervosa in comparison to control families. Int J Eat Disord. 2008;41:37–46.
43. Swartz L. Anorexia nervosa as a culture-bound syndrome. Soc Sci Med. 1985;20:725–730.
44. Keel PK, Klump KL. Are eating disorders culture-bound syndromes? Implications for conceptualizing their etiology. Psychol Bull. 2003;129:747–769
45. Nasser M, Katzman MA, Gordon RA, editors. Eating disorders and cultures in transition. London: Brunner-Routledge; 2001.
46. Garner DM, Vitousek KM, Pike KM. Cognitive behavioral therapy for anorexia nervosa. In: Garner DM. Garfinkel PW, editors. Handbook of clinical treatments in eating disorders. New York: Guilford Press; 1997:94–144.
47. Venkat R, Ogden H. Advertising-induced social comparison and body-image satisfaction: The moderating role of gender, self-esteem and locus of control. J Consum Satisfact Dissatisfact Complain Behav. 2002;15:51–67.
48. Rouleau CR, von Ranson KM. Potential risks of pro-eating disorder websites. Clin Psychol Rev. 2011;31:525–531.
49. Powell LH, Shahabi L, Thoresen CE. Religion and spirituality: Linkages to physical health. Am Psychol. 2003;58:36–52.
50. Gluck ME, Geliebter A. Body image and eating behaviors in Orthodox and Secular Jewish women. J Gender Spec Med. 2002;5:19–24.
51. Allport GW, Ross JM. Personal religion orientation and prejudice. J Person Soc Psychol. 1967;5:432–443.
52. Smith MH, Richards PS, Maglio CJ. Examining the relationship between religious orientation and eating disturbances. Eat Behav. 2004;5:171–180.

Part I
Medical Issues

Chapter 1
The Relationship Between Binge Eating and Attention Deficit Hyperactivity Disorder

Allan S. Kaplan, Andrew L. Howlett, Zeynep Yilmaz and Robert Levitan

Abstract The purpose of this chapter is to review the literature on the relationship between attention-deficit-hyperactivity-disorder (ADHD) and binge eating as seen in bulimia nervosa (BN) and binge eating disorder (BED), including the shared phenomenology, genetics and treatment. The authors reviewed all the published peer reviewed literature in the past decade available through PubMed on the epidemiology, phenomenology, genetics and management of binge eating behavior, especially as it manifests in eating disorders (BN, BED), as well as in obesity and within the context of ADHD throughout the lifespan. It was found that there is a significant association between ADHD and binge eating in clinical populations. Inattentiveness and impulsivity noted in ADHD are thought to play a role in the preoccupations, urges and impulsive behaviors of those who experience binge-eating episodes. Molecular genetic studies have also identified common genes involved in dopamine transport, suggesting a shared genetic predisposition to binge eating, obesity and ADHD. Case reports on individuals with BN and ADHD suggest benefit from psychostimulant medication. In addition, other anti-ADHD medications such as atomoxetine have been used independently in trials to treat obesity and BED. Individuals with current symptoms or a past history of ADHD are at risk of having coexisting binge eating and obesity. Screening for ADHD in patients with binge-eating behaviors may identify individuals who could benefit

A.S. Kaplan (✉)
Center for Addiction and Mental Health, 250 College St Room 832,
Toronto, ON M5T 1R8, Canada
e-mail: allan_kaplan@camh.net

A.S. Kaplan
Center for Addiction and Mental Health, Toronto, Canada

A.S. Kaplan · A.L. Howlett · R. Levitan
Department of Psychiatry, University of Toronto, Toronto, Canada

Z. Yilmaz
University of North Carolina, Chapel Hill, North Carolina, USA

R. Levitan
Mood and Anxiety Program, Center for Addiction and Mental Health, Toronto, Canada

Y. Latzer and D. Stein (eds.), *Bio-Psycho-Social Contributions to Understanding Eating Disorders*, DOI 10.1007/978-3-319-32742-6_1

from anti-ADHD medications. Further research may help to identify shared neurobiological mechanisms and particular risk factors, as well as to determine the efficacy and tolerability of certain medications in this population.

Introduction

Binge eating is defined in Diagnostic and Statistical Manual (DSM 5) as consuming an excessive amount of food in a realtively short period of time [1]. Binge eating at a regular frequency is a phenomenon associated with the three eating disorders recognized by the DSM-5 anorexia nervosa (AN)—binge purge subtype, bulimia nervosa (BN) and binge eating disorder (BED) [1]. Binge eating may also be present in children or adults who are overweight or obese but who do not meet the full criteria for a formal eating disorder such as BED.

Associated with obesity and binge eating disorders are a number of comordid conditions including mood, anxiety and substance use disorders. More recently a relationship between binge eating and both childhood and adult attention deficit-hyperactivity disorder (ADHD) has been noted [2–12].

Adult ADHD is defined by the same criteria as childhood ADHD in the DSM 5; however, the accepted age of onset, on patient recall, is twelve years rather than seven [3, 13]. Individuals evaluated and treated for ADHD in their adult years may or may not have previously been diagnosed with ADHD. It is hypothesized that symptoms of ADHD such as inattentiveness and impulsivity may play a role in the preoccupations, urges and impulsive behaviors of individuals who binge eat [5, 7, 8, 10]. ADHD may also contribute to the development and sustainability of excessive weight gain, for example, the difficulties in maintaining weight loss strategies.

The aim of this paper is to review the association between ADHD and binge eating, weight gain, BED and BN throughout the lifespan. This will include the prevalence as well as similarities noted in phenomenology and molecular genetics between ADHD and binge eating. The management of individuals with these coexisting conditions is also discussed as it may have a significant impact on the treatment of eating disorders and obesity.

Epidemiology

In the US the estimated lifetime prevalence of BN and BED is 1.5 and 3.5 % in women and 0.5 and 2.0 % in men respectively [14]. In 2004 the prevalence of "at-risk-for-overweight" [Body mass index (BMI) > of 85–95 percentile] and "overweight" (BMI > 95 percentile) in children age 2 to 19 in the US was 33.6 and 17.1 % respectively [15]. The same study determined overweight (BMI 25.0–29.9) and obesity (BMI > 30.0) rates in adults as 70.8 and 31.1 % respectively. Obesity has significant costs to individual and public health. In 1998 the estimated cost attributed to both overweight and obesity in the US was $78.5 billion [16].

Initially thought of as a childhood disorder, ADHD is now considered to affect individuals throughout their lifespan. It is estimated to have a lifetime rate of 6–9 % in children, with 70 % persistence into adolescence and 10–60 % persistence into adulthood [17]. The United States National Comorbidity Survey estimates a 4.4 % rate of ADHD in adults [18].

Only one known study has assessed ADHD symptoms and abnormal eating behaviors in the general population [19]. In a cross-sectional analysis Davis et al. evaluated 110 healthy women ages 25–46 for childhood ADHD symptoms and abnormal eating behaviors [19]. Using structural equation modeling the authors found that ADHD symptoms recalled in childhood significantly predicted abnormal eating behaviors including binge eating [19].

The coexisting prevalence of these disorders has been studied in clinical settings. Populations with obesity or an eating disorder have been assessed for symptoms of ADHD [2, 3, 7] and groups of children and adults with ADHD have been assessed for weight gain and eating disorders [11, 20, 21].

(a) Assessing for ADHD in patients with binge eating and/or obesity

In one of two studies involving hospitalized morbidly obese children (BMI > 97 percentile), Cortese et al. aimed to evaluate the association between ADHD and bulimia behaviors in 99 medication-free children by assessing the Connors Parent Rating Scale (CPRS) and the Bulimic Investigatory Test, Edinburgh (BITE) scores [7]. Only mean scores were given and the actual prevalence of ADHD was not provided. The multiple regression analysis controlling for depression (Beck Depression Inventory) and anxiety (State-Trait Anxiety Inventory for Children) scores, identified a significant correlation between CPRS and BITE [7]. In the second study by Agranat-Meged et al., actual prevalence of ADHD was determined. Of 26 morbidly obese children, 10 boys and 5 girls (57.7 %) were identified as meeting the criteria for a diagnosis of ADHD (6 had inattentive type and 9 had the combined type) [2]. The significant ADHD symptomatology and the increased prevalence of ADHD demonstrated in these two clinical samples of morbidly obese children may not reflect the true incidence in overweight and obese children in the general population.

In a chart review of 215 adults (193 women and 22 men) seeking treatment for obesity, 27 % (50 women and 9 men) met full criteria for ADHD-Inattentive type by structured interviews using DSM IV criteria [3]. No information on actual eating behaviors was provided and no subjects diagnosed with ADHD were on anti-ADHD medications. In the group with a BMI > 40 kg/m^2, 42.6 % had ADHD. In addition, weight reduction during treatment was significantly lower in obese adults with ADHD compared to obese participants who had no evidence of ADHD. In this study, comorbidities were not controlled for, and given that mood and anxiety disorders are more common in those with ADHD and obesity than in individuals without ADHD or of normal weight, these confounders could also contribute to maximum BMI.

(b) Assessing for binge eating and obesity in populations with ADHD
The prevalence of obesity was assessed in two studies of children with ADHD [11, 20]. Curtin et al. reviewed the charts of 98 children with ADHD; the determined prevalence of "at-risk-for-overweight" was 29 % and the prevalence of "overweight" was 17.3 % [20]. There were no differences in the prevalence of either category compared to the NHANES study [20]. Of the 32 children on anti-ADHD medication, only 5 were "at-risk-for-overweight" and 2 were considered "overweight", both rates being significantly lower compared to the group of ADHD children not on medication [20]. No individual on medication was underweight, compared to 5 underweight individuals who were not on medication [20]. This study represents a population identified at a tertiary clinic and may not be representative of ADHD and its relationship with overweight in the general community.

The other study included 97 German boys with a mean age of 10 years and all with ADHD-combined type [11]. No comorbidy was present, with the exception of conduct disorder, found in 58 % of the participants. The authors hypothesized that symptoms of hyperactivity would predict a lower weight compared to a young population without ADHD. To their surprise, the mean BMI–SDS in this group was significantly higher than mean reference value. Specifically, 19.6 % of these participants were overweight and 7.2 % obese, significantly higher than expected for this age-group in Germany.

More recently, Biederman et al. performed a case-control study to assess whether girls with ADHD were more at risk for developing eating disorders (AN and BN) [21]. 123 Caucasian girls with ADHD from two hospital based settings were compared to 122 Caucasian controls from a list of outpatients. The girls were assessed at baseline (ages 6–18) and again approximately 5-years later (ages 10–25) for a history or current presentation of symptoms of AN and/or BN. Assessments were blindly rated and a diagnosis of an eating disorder was made if at least half of the relevant DSM-IV criteria were met. Unfortunately, those meeting full criteria were not differentiated for the final analysis. After 5-years and including all assessments, 20 (16 %) girls with ADHD had an eating disorder (6 AN, 10 BN, 4 reported both AN and BN). In the non-ADHD group, 5 (5 %) had an eating disorder (3 AN, 2BN). Females with ADHD were more than three times more likely to meet partial or full criteria for an eating disorder, more than five times more likely to meet criteria for BN and more than twice more likely to meet criteria for AN. This is the first study that demonstrates a potential relationship between ADHD and AN in children and adolescents; however this finding may be an over representation, given that the authors included also cases when full criteria were not met, and most details were provided by recall.

In two separate case-cohort studies of adults with and without ADHD, Surman et al. reported that women with ADHD (the majority had inattentive type) had an incidence of BN in 11 and 12 %, respectively, compared to 1 and 3 %, respectively in women of the non ADHD group ($p < 0.05$); the incidence of BN in men was negligible [12].

In Brazil, Mattos et al. evaluated 86 adults with ADHD for BED and discovered an incidence of 8.3 %, much higher than in the general population [22]. As expected, patients with ADHD and BED had significantly higher rates of comorbid psychiatric disorders, including depression and anxiety, compared to those with ADHD but without BED.

The relationship between ADHD and obesity is evident in clinical populations. In particular, boys with ADHD certainly appear to be at risk for obesity [2]; however, in adolescence and adulthood, women with ADHD, more so than men, are likely to present with BED and BN [12]. It is unclear whether the prevalence of ADHD in individuals seeking weight loss treatment is greater or less than in those who do not seek weight loss treatment.

Phenomenology

The significant coexistence of ADHD and BN, BED and obesity in prevalence studies leads to many hypotheses about the unique and shared characteristics of these disorders [2–12]. Traditionally, ADHD has its onset in childhood, which suggests that it precedes BED and BN that are typically disorders of adolescents and adults. In addition, certain features of ADHD may affect the eating behaviors and outcomes of men and women differently. When comparing younger children (10 years and younger) to older children (11 years and older), the prevalence of all ADHD subtypes may decrease with age for both males and females, with the exception of "inattentive" symptoms, which are increased in older females [23]. It has also been hypothesized that gender may dictate how a biologic vulnerability is expressed, based on cultural and hormone influences leading to the presentation of different symptoms at different times in the life cycle [24].

Although girls with ADHD have been shown to have a higher risk of developing BN than girls with no ADHD [12], there are no established features of ADHD that may put a person at a greater risk of developing an eating disorder. Common symptoms of ADHD, BN and BED include impulsivity, poor affect regulation, lack of self-awareness and low self-esteem [2, 7]. Impulsivity is thought to be a common characteristic of individuals with ADHD and BN, including risk-taking behaviors such as self-harm, promiscuity and substance use.

The inattentiveness seen in ADHD may be harder to appreciate in eating disorders, although it may contribute to preoccupations with food and body image and related urges to binge and purge. Schweickert suggests that compulsive eating may be a compensatory mechanism to help individuals control the frustration associated with attention and organizational difficulties [25]. In a case series of six subjects with BN and comorbid ADHD, all diagnosed with the inattentive subtype [26], their bingeing and purging behaviors have been primarily associated with their impulsivity. Following treatment for their ADHD, all cases have reported the cessation of the desire to binge or purge, a finding related by the authors to an improvement in attention span rather than a decrease in impulsivity [7].

Davis et al. have suggested that deficient inhibitory control including poor planning for the future and a failure to monitor one's behavior effectively can lead to over-eating, and difficulty in maintaining dietary strategies [8]. For example, when faced with a choice between immediacy and delay—even if the latter will provide greater rewards—individuals with ADHD will typically opt for the immediate choice. Fast food, which is often of high caloric content, may be required to satisfy these urges immediately, its choice also being the consequence of a strong delay aversion.

While there is a strong association between ADHD and binge eating, not all cases of ADHD develop comorbid illnesses such as obesity, BED and BN. Of equal importance is to understand why this occurs, and what protective factors may exist. For instance, it has yet to be determined whether or not children or adolescents treated adequately for ADHD are less likely to develop obesity, BED or BN; nevertheless, in the study by Holtcamp et al. [11], fewer boys on psychostimulant medication were overweight than those not treated.

Genetics

A number of studies using molecular genetics have identified vulnerable genes in subjects with ADHD as well as in those with binge eating, obesity and BN. Several candidate genes reported to be associated with ADHD, including dopaminergic genes such as DRD4, DAT1, DRD5, DBH, and serotonergic genes such as 5HTT and HTR1B, have also been shown to be associated with binge eating, maximum weight gain and BN [27–29].

(a) DRD4

The DRD4 gene encodes for a dopamine receptor on the postsynaptic neuron. Only one study known to date has explored the association of DRD4 in subjects assessed for ADHD and its relationship to weight [27]. Levitan et al. have discovered that a subset of women with seasonal affective disorder have had the 7-repeat allele of DRD4, this gene being significantly associated with both maximum lifetime BMI and ADHD symptoms [27]. The 7R allele of the DRD4 is associated with a decreased affinity for dopamine in postsynaptic neurons [30] and is also associated with ADHD [31, 32]. The same gene has also been found in 55 women (34 %) with BN, being significantly linked to a high maximum lifetime BMI [28]. Recently, the same allele has been found to predict the presence of childhood ADHD in adult subjects with BN [29].

(b) DAT

The dopamine transporter (DAT) of the presynaptic neuron is known to be a key regulator of dopamine, and recent genetic and treatment studies have highlighted the role of DAT independently in binge eating [19, 30] and in ADHD [33]. In the case of the DAT1 gene, there appears to be a difference in the expression of either the short [7] or [9] or long [10, 11] allele of the 3′ untranscribed region (UTR) of the variable number tandem repeat (VNTR) polymorphism amongst those with binge eating. In a group of 90 female Japanese patients who had an eating disorder with binge eating behavior, the frequency of the short allele was significantly higher compared to the control group [30]. Similarly, Davis et al. assessed DAT1 genotype differences on appetite ratings to a snack-food cue in subjects with BED and healthy age-matched controls [19]. Subjects with BED and at least one copy of the 9-repeat allele showed a significant suppression of appetite in response to methylphenidate compared with controls with this short allele. In addition, the drug response for methylphenidate was indistinguishable from placebo in all subjects with the 10/10 genotype, irrespective of diagnosis.

As for ADHD, DAT1 has been investigated as a primary candidate gene because stimulant medications are known to bind to the DAT, inhibiting reuptake and increasing synaptic dopamine [34]. An association between ADHD and the 10-repeat allele has been demonstrated in a number of studies, although not in all [35]. In addition, both the 9 and 10 alleles of the DAT1 gene have been examined in a number of pharmacogenetic studies in an attempt to predict response to methylphenidate. There are inconsistent results amongst these studies, which are often limited by sample size, short-term outcomes and the use of different methodologies [35].

(c) Gene-Gene Interactions

Despite the fact that certain genotypes are significantly associated with ADHD, binge eating or both, such vulnerable genes are not present in all cases, and may be also present in those without these disorders. This genetic variability suggests the likelihood of more complex gene-gene interactions. For example, a more exclusive and currently unknown genetic variant that is overrepresented in individuals with BED may interact with DAT1 to suppress appetite in response to stimulation administration [19]. Other potential gene-gene interactions include brain-derived neurotrophic factor (BDNF) and the 7R allele of DRD4 [28]. In their molecular study of women with BN, Kaplan et al. established that there was no main effect of the BDNF gene in predicting maximal BMI in individuals with BN; however, the BDNF Met66 allele did interact with the 7R allele of DRD4 to promote high lifetime BMI [28]. This could reflect a direct interaction between the two genes under consideration and/or their gene products and/or a deleterious effect of low BDNF expression on the early development of key dopamine neurons such as in the mesocorticolimbic pathway.

Treatment

The literature on the treatment of comorbid binge eating and ADHD is lacking; however the common approach has been to use anti-ADHD medications such as psychostimulants to treat this coexisting condition. Psychostimulants are the first line agent for ADHD and are one of the most efficacious psychiatric medications.

There have been no randomized controlled trials (RCT) evaluating the effectiveness of psychostimulant medication for comorbid ADHD and binge eating. Lisdexamfetamine (Vyvanse) has now received FDA approval for the treatment of BED; however, in the RCT that lead to FDA approval, subjects with comorbid BED and ADHD were excluded from this trial [36]. There have been case reports of successful treatment with psychostimulants for both symptoms of ADHD and binge eating [24–26, 37]. These studies are reviewed below.

(a) Methylphenidate
The most common treatment of ADHD is the use of psychostimulants such as methylphenidate (MPH). Initially prescribed as immediate-release dosing, multiple versions of controlled release are now available. Controlled release tablets are becoming more commonly used and have shown to be safer, more convenient and more efficacious [17, 38, 39]. MPH is a dopamine reuptake inhibitor, which increases brain synaptic dopamine and improves concentration, attention and other cognitive symptoms associated with ADHD. It also has been shown to suppress appetite. The short-term effect of MPH on energy intake was investigated in two double-blind laboratory studies. Ong et al. used methylphenidate (IV) or placebo blindly in 8 cases of BN and discovered a very rapid suppression of bulimic symptoms including self-ratings of hunger and amount of food eaten [40]. Leddy et al. used short-acting MPH in 9 obese adult males to assess for changes in energy intake [41]. All subjects had similar hunger scores before ingesting either a placebo or a moderate dose (0.5 mg/kg) or a high dose (1.0 mg/kg) of MPH. Participants consumed 34 % fewer kilocalories of pizza after ingesting the moderate dose of MPH; there was no statistical significant difference between the moderate and high dose of MPH.

There are a number of case reports using MPH to treat individuals with BN and symptoms or full diagnosis of ADHD. Dukarm et al. studied the treatment of 6 individuals (5 female, 1 male) between the ages of 16–24 who were all diagnosed with BN by the age of 16 and then later diagnosed with ADHD—Inattentive type [26]. Some were noted to have impulsivity but no symptoms of hyperactivity were recalled. One individual had been suffering for nine-years with bingeing and purging. A positive response was found in all 6 cases following the use of dextroamphetamine. This was evident in a decrease in the desire to binge, and in food- and body-image related anxiety, and in improved attention and mood. A few relapses were reported when the patients occasionally forgot to take their medication.

Other case reports show similar effects of short-acting psychostimulants. Schweickert et al. report a case of a 25 year old female with ADHD—hyperactive-impulsive subtype who would binge and purge in times of stress up to 5 times per day [25]. Once she entered college she became overwhelmed, having difficulties with distractibility, concentration, retaining information, organizing and feeling restless and as a consequence she began bingeing and purging [25]. With the initiation of MPH she had complete cessation of binges attributed to improved concentration, decreased restlessness and distractibility while her appetite remained unaffected [25].

Drimmer et al. reports 3 cases of treating binge eating with MPH, 2 of who also had ADHD diagnosed as adults and the other case had comorbid major depressive disorder and PTSD [37]. All cases had significant improvement with a few relapses spanning over two years. The main reason for relapse was reported as forgetting to take the medication and acting on the urge to binge and or purge.

Sokol et al. reported on 2 cases of BN, one with ADHD and the other with cluster B personality disorder (i.e. impulsive, unstable affect and inattentive) who also scored high on the Connors Rating Scale (for symptoms of ADHD) [24]. Both cases had significant improvement in their symptoms; one case had complete cessation of her binging and purging whereas the other case had a significant reduction in binge episodes and in her Connors score [24].

(b) Atomoxetine

Atomoxetine, a second-line agent for ADHD, was also used recently in two RCTs to treat women with obesity [42] and adults with BED [43]. There are no studies or reports of its use in treating individuals with ADHD and a comorbid eating disorder. In a 12-week RCT, 15 of 30 women received atomoxetine therapy starting at 25 mg/day orally with a gradual increase to 100 mg/day over 1 week with an identical placebo dosing for the remaining 15 participants [44]. Counseling was minimal with a 10-min monthly session from a dietician and body weight in kilograms was the primary outcome. Atomoxetine demonstrated modest albeit statistically significant short-term weight loss relative to placebo (−3.6 kg vs. 0.1 kg). McElroy et al. studied the efficacy of atomoxetine (40–120 mg) in a 10-week, double-blinded RCT of outpatients with BED [43]. The primary outcome was binge episode frequency with a number of related secondary outcomes. The binge episode frequency was significantly lower in the atomoxetine group compared to placebo. Among the secondary measures, a number of scales were administered throughout the study; although a measurement of ADHD symptoms was not employed.

In both studies, side effects appeared to be more common with atomoxetine than with placebo, but were generally well tolerated. However some participants withdrew early because of adverse events including tachycardia, depression, constipation and nervousness. There were no significant differences between treatment groups with regard to changes in blood pressure and heart rate and in mean change from baseline to final visit for fasting insulin, triglycerides and cholesterol in both studies.

Future Directions

The evidence of an association between binge eating behavior and ADHD in terms of shared phenomenology, molecular genetics and response to treatment provides a foundation for further research. The investigations of gene-gene and gene-environment interactions in subjects with both ADHD and BED or BN will not only provide a better understanding of this relationship and associated risk factors but may also help predict response with medications.

Further studies are also needed to determine the efficacy, safety and tolerability of using psychostimulants for individuals with both symptoms of ADHD and binge eating, including those with BN or BED. Safety concerns using instant release psychostimulants include side effects such as increased blood pressure and heart rate, weight loss, as well as the potential for misuse in this somewhat impulsive population. Instant-release forms of psychostimulants have been associated with higher and more rapid dopamine peaks and consequently, mild euphoric states and rebound effects and thus carry greater potential for misuse. The recent availability of controlled release long acting psychostimulants has been shown to reduce the incidence of such side effects and thereby reduce the potential for misuse and tolerance [45]. This drug delivery system is now preferred in the treatment of ADHD [46] and provides a safe alternative worth studying in those with ADHD and BN or BED.

The evidence presented in this review supports the importance of and need for clinical screening for symptoms of ADHD and binge eating, when indicated, throughout the lifespan, especially in individuals who are overweight or obese. The current most effective treatment for individuals with BN and BED is cognitive behavior therapy. While psycho-education and psychotherapy are used in patients with ADHD, the most effective treatment is psychostimulants. The exact role of cognitive behavior therapy and psychostimulants when both conditions coexist remains to be investigated. However, a logical next step would be to evaluate the effectiveness of long acting psychotimulants for subjects with both ADHD and binge eating through a rigorously conducted randomized placebo controlled trial.

Take Home Points

- A significant association may exist between ADHD and binge eating in clinical populations.
- Therefore it is of importance to do a clinical screening for both symptoms of ADHD and binge eating, in individuals who are overweight or obese throughout the lifespan.
- Inattentivess and impulsivity noted in ADHD are thought to play a key role in the preoccupations, urges and impulsive behaviors of individuals experiencing binge-eating episodes.
- Molecular genetic studies have identified common genes involved in dopamine transport, suggesting a shared genetic predisposition to binge eating, obesity and ADHD.
- Case reports on individuals with BN and ADHD suggest reduction in bingeing behaviors, and hence also in purging behaviors with psychostimulant medication.
- Psychostimulants and other mediations treating ADHD such as atomoxetine may be used in the treatment of ADHD patients with concurrent BED-related obesity.
- Further research may help to identify shared neurobiological mechanisms and particular risk factors, as well as to determine the efficacy and tolerability of certain medications in individuals with combined ADHD and EDs/obesity.

References

1. American Psychiatric Association. Diagnostic and statistical manual of mental disorders. 4th ed. Text revision. Washington, DC: American Psychiatric Association; 2000.
2. Agranat-Meged AN, Deitcher C, Goldzweig G, Leibenson L, Stein M, Galili-Weisstub E. Childhood obesity and attention deficit/hyperactivity disorder: a newly described comorbidity in obese hospitalized children. Int J Eat Disord. 2005;37:357–9.
3. Altfas JR. Prevalence of attention deficit/hyperactivity disorder among adults in obesity treatment. BMC Psychiatry. 2002;13(2):9.
4. Bazar KA, Yun AJ, Lee PY, Daniel SM, Doux JD. Obesity and ADHD may represent different manifestations of a common environmental oversampling syndrome: a model for revealing mechanistic overlap among cognitive, metabolic, and inflammatory disorders. Med Hypotheses. 2006;66:263–9.
5. Cortese S, Bernardina BD, Mouren MC. Attention-deficit/hyperactivity disorder (ADHD) and binge eating. Nutr Rev. 2007;65:404–11.
6. Cortese S, Isnard P, Dalla Bernardina B, Mouren MC. Attention-deficit/hyperactivity disorder, binge eating, and obesity. J Clin Psychiatry. 2007;68:976; author's reply 976–7.
7. Cortese S, Isnard P, Frelut ML, Michel G, Quantin L, Guedeney A, et al. Association between symptoms of attention-deficit/hyperactivity disorder and bulimic behaviors in a clinical sample of severely obese adolescents. Int J Obes (Lond.). 2007;31:340–6.
8. Davis C, Levitan RD, Smith M, Tweed S, Curtis C. Associations among overeating, overweight, and attention deficit/hyperactivity disorder: a structural equation modeling approach. Eat Behav. 2006;7:266–74.
9. Ersson G, Klanger AR, Wallsten T, Nilsson KW, Lindstrom L. Possible connection between eating disorders and ADHD. Bulimia can relieve ADHD symptoms, central nervous stimulants are of good help. Lakartidningen. 2007;104:1402–5.
10. Fleming J, Lance L. ADHD and disordered eating. In: Quinn P, Nadeau K, eds. Gender issues and ADHD: research, diagnosis, and treatment: Advantage Books; 2002.
11. Holtkamp K, Konrad K, Muller B, Heussen N, Herpertz S, Herpertz-Dahlmann B, et al. Overweight and obesity in children with Attention-Deficit/Hyperactivity Disorder. Int J Obes Relat Metab Disord. 2004;28:685–9.
12. Surman CB, Randall ET, Biederman J. Association between attention-deficit/hyperactivity disorder and bulimia nervosa: analysis of 4 case-control studies. J Clin Psychiatry. 2006;67:351–4.
13. Faraone SV, Biederman J, Spencer T, Mick E, Murray K, Petty C, et al. Diagnosing adult attention deficit hyperactivity disorder: are late onset and subthreshold diagnoses valid? Am J Psychiatry. 2006;163:1720–9.
14. Hudson JI, Hiripi E, Pope HG Jr, Kessler RC. The prevalence and correlates of eating disorders in the National Comorbidity Survey Replication. Biol Psychiatry. 2007;61:348–58.
15. Ogden CL, Carroll MD, Curtin LR, McDowell MA, Tabak CJ, Flegal KM. Prevalence of overweight and obesity in the United States, 1999–2004. JAMA. 2006;295:1549–55.
16. Finkelstein EA, Fiebelkorn IC, Wang G. National medical spending attributable to overweight and obesity: how much, and who's paying? Health Aff. (Millwood) 2003;Suppl Web Exclusives (W3):219–26.
17. Wender PH, Wolf LE, Wasserstein J. Adults with ADHD. An overview. Ann NY Acad Sci. 2001;931:1–16.
18. Kessler RC, Adler L, Barkley R, Biederman J, Conners CK, Demler O, et al. The prevalence and correlates of adult ADHD in the united states: results from the national comorbidity survey replication. Am J Psychiatry. 2006;163:716–23.
19. Davis C, Levitan RD, Kaplan AS, Carter J, Reid C, Curtis C, et al. Dopamine transporter gene (DAT1) associated with appetite suppression to methylphenidate in a case-control study of binge eating disorder. Neuropsychopharmacology. 2007;32:2199–206.

20. Curtin C, Bandini LG, Perrin EC, Tybor DJ, Must A. Prevalence of overweight in children and adolescents with attention deficit hyperactivity disorder and autism spectrum disorders: a chart review. BMC Pediatr. 2005;5:48.
21. Biederman J, Ball SW, Monuteaux MC, Surman CB, Johnson JL, Zeitlin S. Are girls with ADHD at risk for eating disorders? Results from a controlled, five-year prospective study. J Dev Behav Pediatr. 2007;28:302–7.
22. Mattos P, Saboya E, Ayrao V, Segenreich D, Duchesne M, Coutinho G. Comorbid eating disorders in a Brazilian attention-deficit/hyperactivity disorder adult clinical sample. Rev Bras Psiquiatr. 2004;26:248–50.
23. Levy F, Hay DA, Bennett KS, McStephen M. Gender differences in ADHD subtype comorbidity. J Am Acad Child Adolesc Psychiatry. 2005;44:368–76.
24. Sokol MS, Gray NS, Goldstein A, Kaye WH. Methylphenidate treatment for bulimia nervosa associated with a cluster B personality disorder. Int J Eat Disord. 1999;25:233–7.
25. Schweickert LA, Strober M, Moskowitz A. Efficacy of methylphenidate in bulimia nervosa comorbid with attention-deficit hyperactivity disorder: a case report. Int J Eat Disord. 1997;21:299–301.
26. Dukarm CP. Bulimia nervosa and attention deficit hyperactivity disorder: a possible role for stimulant medication. J Women's Health (Larchmt). 2005;14:345–50.
27. Levitan RD, Masellis M, Basile VS, Lam RW, Kaplan AS, Davis C, et al. The dopamine-4 receptor gene associated with binge eating and weight gain in women with seasonal affective disorder: an evolutionary perspective. Biol Psychiatry. 2004;56:665–9.
28. Kaplan AS, Levitan RD, Yilmaz Z, Davis C, Tharmalingam S, Kennedy JL. A DRD4/BDNF gene-gene interaction associated with maximum BMI in women with bulimia nervosa. Int J Eat Disord. 2008;41:22–8.
29. Kaplan AS, Levitan R, Tharmalingam S, Yilmaz Z, Kennedy J. Bulimia Nervosa and ADHD: Shared phenomenology, psychometrics and genetics. Presented at the annual meeting of the Eating Disorder Research Society, Oct 2007, Pittsburgh Pa.
30. Shinohara M, Mizushima H, Hirano M, Shioe K, Nakazawa M, Hiejima Y, et al. Eating disorders with binge-eating behavior are associated with the s allele of the 3'-UTR VNTR polymorphism of the dopamine transporter gene. J Psychiatry Neurosci. 2004;29:134–7.
31. Asghari V, Sanyal S, Buchwaldt S, Paterson A, Jovanovic V, Van Tol HH. Modulation of intracellular cyclic AMP levels by different human dopamine D4 receptor variants. J Neurochem. 1995;65:1157–65.
32. Gornick MC, Addington A, Shaw P, Bobb AJ, Sharp W, Greenstein D, et al. Association of the dopamine receptor D4 (DRD4) gene 7-repeat allele with children with attention-deficit/hyperactivity disorder (ADHD): an update. Am J Med Genet B. Neuropsychiatr Genet 2007;144:379–82.
33. Elia J, Devoto M. ADHD genetics: 2007 update. Curr Psychiatry Rep. 2007;9:434–9.
34. Volkow ND, Fowler JS, Wang G, Ding Y, Gatley SJ. Mechanism of action of methylphenidate: insights from PET imaging studies. J Atten Disord. 2002;6(Suppl. 1): S31–43.
35. Stein MA, Waldman ID, Sarampote CS, Seymour KE, Robb AS, Conlon C, et al. Dopamine transporter genotype and methylphenidate dose response in children with ADHD. Neuropsychopharmacology. 2005;30:1374–82.
36. McElroy S, Hudson J, Ferreira-Cornwell C, et al. Lisdexafetamine dimesylate for adults with modertae to severe binge eating disorder: results of two pivotal phase 3 randomized controlled trials. Neuropsychopharmacology. 2015;4:1251–1260.
37. Drimmer EJ. Stimulant treatment of bulimia nervosa with and without attention-deficit disorder: three case reports. Nutrition. 2003;19:76–7.
38. Biederman J, Faraone SV, Spencer TJ, Mick E, Monuteaux MC, Aleardi M. Functional impairments in adults with self-reports of diagnosed ADHD: a controlled study of 1001 adults in the community. J Clin Psychiatry. 2006;67:524–40.

39. Medori R, Ramos-Quiroga JA, Casas M, Kooij JJ, Niemela A, Trott GE, et al. A randomized, placebo-controlled trial of three fixed dosages of prolonged-release OROS methylphenidate in adults with attention-deficit/hyperactivity disorder. Biol Psychiatry. 2008;63:981–9.
40. Ong YL, Checkley SA, Russell GF. Suppression of bulimic symptoms with methylamphetamine. Br J Psychiatry. 1983;143:288–93.
41. Leddy JJ, Epstein LH, Jaroni JL, Roemmich JN, Paluch RA, Goldfield GS, et al. Influence of methylphenidate on eating in obese men. Obes Res. 2004;12:224–32.
42. Gadde KM, Yonish GM, Wagner HR 2nd, Foust MS, Allison DB. Atomoxetine for weight reduction in obese women: a preliminary randomized controlled trial. Int J Obes (Lond.). 2006;30:1138–42.
43. McElroy SL, Guerdjikova A, Kotwal R, Welge JA, Nelson EB, Lake KA, et al. Atomoxetine in the treatment of binge-eating disorder: a randomized placebo-controlled trial. J Clin Psychiatry. 2007;68:390–8.
44. Gadde KM, Yonish GM, Wagner HR 2nd, Foust MS, Allison DB. Atomoxetine for weight reduction in obese women: a preliminary randomized controlled trial. Int J Obes (Lond.). 2006;30:1138–42.
45. Goksoyr PK, Nottestad JA. The burden of untreated ADHD among adults: The role of stimulant medication. Addict Behav. 2008;33:342–6.
46. Davidson MA. ADHD in adults: A review of the literature. J Atten Disord. 2007;11:628–41.

Chapter 2
The Interplay Between Eating and Sleeping Behavior in Adolescence: Normative and Disordered Trajectories

Yael Latzer, Sarah L. Weinberger-Litman, Leib Litman and Orna Tzicshinsky

Abstract The present chapter deals with the relation between eating and sleeping patterns among adolescents. The first part describes both normative and pathological changes in eating and sleeping behavior. In the second part, studies that examine sleep-wake patterns among adolescents suffering from eating disorders are presented. Finally, the importance of maintaining a balance between adolescents' needs for autonomy and the supervision and support of parents as providers of healthy nutrition and sleeping habits is discussed.

Introduction

The present chapter deals with the relation between eating and sleeping patterns in adolescence. Adolescence is an age of significant and constant transitions and change. Eating and sleeping habits at this age reach a critical juncture in which familiar childhood patterns become completely transformed. Most of these modifications are normative. Therefore, it is important to separate them from pathological eating and sleeping patterns. The connection between changes in sleeping and eating behavior is particularly pronounced among adolescents [1, 2].

Y. Latzer (✉)
Faculty of Social Welfare and Health Sciences, Haifa University, Mount Carmel, Haifa, Israel
e-mail: latzery@gmail.com

Y. Latzer
Eating Disorders Institute, Rambam Medical Center, Haifa, Israel

S.L. Weinberger-Litman
Department of Psychology, Marymount Manhattan College, New York, USA

L. Litman
Department of Psychology, Lander College, New York, USA

O. Tzicshinsky
Behavioral Science Department, Emek Yezreel Academic College, Emek Yezreel, Israel

Y. Latzer and D. Stein (eds.), *Bio-Psycho-Social Contributions to Understanding Eating Disorders*, DOI 10.1007/978-3-319-32742-6_2

Changes in Eating and Sleeping Behaviors During Puberty

Adolescence is an age with a series of continuous dramatic transitions and adjustments on the physiological, neuroendocrine, psychological, developmental, and cognitive level. It is also a time of significant change in the social and family environment. Beyond physiological growth and development, the two major objectives during adolescence are independence and identity construction.

In the last few decades, researchers have divided the adolescence period into three separate age-based developmental stages: 12–13, 14–15, and 16–18 [3]. Each developmental stage present changes in eating and sleeping patterns in accordance with the physiological and psychological changes taking place [4].

Eating and sleeping habits reach a critical stage when familiar childhood patterns significantly change. In contrast to their childhood eating behavior, adolescents tend to eat more during puberty and to adapt new eating habits, such as eating at different hours of the day or changing taste preferences. In a similar manner, adolescents' sleep patterns within a 24-h period typically change as well. Even though adolescents require approximately 9 h of sleep a night, they seldom reach that requirement [4–7]. Most changes in eating and sleeping during adolescence are normative, therefore, it is essential to separate them from pathological patterns. Nonetheless, the way in which adolescents eat and sleep is related to their genetic predisposition, personality structure and life tempo, as well as their social and cultural environment [7]. Almost half of adolescents adopt regular and appropriate eating and sleeping habits and respond in an adequate way to age-related demands. However, approximately 10 % of all adolescents have difficulty in adjusting to changes. Although their adverse response to new or frustrating situations may be apparent even before they reach adolescence, their inflexibility intensifies during this period. Some adolescents react to hunger signals with great intensity and ask to eat immediately when they feel hungry, while others will be able to wait patiently for the food to be prepared. In addition, there are adolescents who enjoy a variety of food, whereas others are picky eaters who are harder to please [8]. Similarly, these features are manifested in sleep behavior patterns. Some adolescents can sleep less and still manage well, while others need more sleep in order to function [9–11]. Whereas some keep strictly to a regular sleep routine, others are more flexible and can adapt their sleep time to their daily activities.

Eating Habits During Puberty: Normative Perspective

The extreme physiological, hormonal, psychological, and cognitive changes that occur during the transition from childhood to adolescence cause meaningful changes in nutrition and eating habits. Adolescence is characterized by an accelerated growth process, resulting in a strong feeling of hunger and a powerful need to eat. At this stage, the responsibility for eating gradually moves from the parents to the adolescents, as parental control decreases. Significant changes occur in adolescents' food intake and choices, as well as in their eating patterns and schedules. Adolescents may begin to experiment with food choices and prepare meals by themselves as they strive for autonomy in all areas of life. These changes and experimentation are part of normal behavior, and forming one's independence on this level leads to the development of new skills in order to reach full food management.

Adolescents tend to gravitate towards different eating behavior and food choices, often experimenting with types of diets, such as vegetarianism [12]. Although they need a balanced diet in order to meet all of their developmental requirements, they often do not choose the appropriate foods and instead consume high-calorie fast foods while eating out with their friends. They are also inclined to avoid family meals and to skip breakfast. Adolescents are profoundly influenced by their peers and by the media, are keen on following the latest trends in nutrition and diet, and are subject to superstitions and myths about eating that have no connection to any proven nutritional quality [13, 14].

The emotional fluctuation typical of adolescence is also manifested in eating behavior.

Emotional eating, which frequently results in dieting and binge eating behavior, is influenced by mood, social events, and social company [15]. Eating late at night is very common and is not necessarily connected to hunger or satiation [16–18]. In addition to radical changes in eating behavior, food preferences also go through changes that may be bizarre and contradict personal taste.

Generally, unrestrained eating behaviors are within the normal range and are not considered to be pathological. They represent an attempt to test limitations, to strengthen a sense of independence, to take risks, and to try new and extreme behaviors. The main difference between pathological and normal eating is that normal eating does not interfere with functioning and is not associated with a loss of control over eating [19–23].

Several changes in eating behaviors and nutrition patterns are characteristic of the transition from childhood to adolescence. These changes include the amount of food eaten, the setting where eating happens, and a less structured eating pattern. Additionally there is an increase in emotional eating, characterized by extreme changes in eating styles and dieting behavior, more frequent eating out. These changes are influenced by a complex combination of psychosocial and physiological factors. Furthermore, it is consistently shown that sleep deprivation in childhood and adolescents is directly associated with changes in food intake [24–26].

Sleep Structure and Habits During Puberty: Normative Perspective

While the specific function(s) of sleep are not precisely clear, it is evident that human beings cannot exist without sleep, and sleep has a multifaceted effect on wakefulness, though its specific function is still not completely clear. Research data show clearly shows that sleep deprivation affects various bodily systems, such as temperature regulation, immune and metabolic functions [27, 28], as well as cognitive performance [11, 29–31] and sensory functions [32]. During the transitions from childhood to adolescence and from adolescence to adulthood, significant changes in sleep patterns and daily sleep-wake cycles occur [4]. Rresearch over the past few decades has shown that the preliminary assumption was incorrect insofar as [33] there are the variety of physiological, affective, and social changes in adolescence that demand almost the same amount of sleep as in childhood [10, 29, 33, 34]. Nevertheless, in contrast with children, adolescents go to sleep much later and experience a significant delay in sleep onset, both during the week and even more so on the weekends [35, 36]. Another previous premise it was previously thought was that adolescents could make up for less sleep time during the week on the weekends. Yet today, this premise is considered only partially correct, and research has shown that there is no satisfactory compensation for sleep deprivation experienced during the week [37].

This sleep deprivation can be attributed to the increased availability of activities and stimuli to which adolescents are exposed, such as media the internet, television, and cell mobile phones, as well as the high expectations from their environment, including academic demands, social activities, sports and other extracurricular activities [7, 24]. However, it has been found that some after-school activities influence sleep patterns more than others. For example, whereas homework only partly influences a later bedtime, extracurricular activities, especially in sports, have a greater influence. In addition, part-time employment after school for those who work more than 19 h a week likewise increases sleep deficiency [7, 38].

Due to the variety of psychosocial factors contributing to sleep deficiency among adolescents, these patterns are found throughout numerous cultures to be universal and multicultural [35, 38–40]. Moreover, they become more pronounced as adolescents mature [41, 42]. One of the most significant factors relating to sleep patterns in adolescence is the extent to which parents supervise bedtime schedules [43]. Research shows that the major change in parental control occurs in the transition from childhood to adolescence. It was found that the more adolescents mature, the lower the parents' influence is on their sleep patterns [43]. Whereas 48–54 % of children between the ages of 10–11 reported that their parents had an influence on their bedtime, only 20–38 % of children between the ages of 12–13 did likewise.

In contrast, regarding wake-up time, it was found that 70 % of adolescents between the ages of 12–13 reported that they woke up with the help of an alarm clock or their parents, as opposed to only 38–46 % of children aged 10–11, who spontaneously woke up earlier. Another influential factor on sleep deficiency during the school week is the early hour of the commencement of school. Several studies conducted in the United States, Israel and in other countries have demonstrated that [44] delaying the school start time by 1 h (from 7:30 to 8:30 a.m.) resulted in 51 more minutes of sleep time and school start times for adolescents increased total sleep and, significantly improves cognitive and school performance and does not did not influence sleep onset time [24, 30, 45]. Similar findings were found in studies conducted in the United States [46].

Regarding Physiological aspects, research has shown that adolescents need an average of 9.25 h of sleep per night, in comparison with children who need an average of 10 h of sleep per night. The maturation of the nervous system in adolescents causes a decrease of approximately 40 % in the slow wave stages 3 and 4 (Delta sleep), as well as a reduction in REM latency and some increase in stages 1 and 2 and wakefulness during the night [4, 47]. The circadian system (physiological changes during a 24-h period) is also is also shortened and fixed on 90 min per sleep cycle [48]. The quantity and intensity of deep sleep (Delta sleep) depends on the wakefulness period before sleep, a factor that points to the influence of homeostatic regulation [49] on the timing of the sleep-wake rhythm during a 24-h period, as well as on the sleep structure in adolescence [5, 47, 49].

Studies on isolation (with no light-darkness indication) or on short sleep-wake cycles (MSLT) over a 24-h period have shown that sleep onset and REM change are the result of daily changes in body temperature or in the melatonin secretion rhythm. Melatonin (5-methoxy-N-acetyltryptamine) is a natural hormone that is produced and secreted from the pineal gland on a fixed 24-h cycle. The secretion of melatonin begins with the onset of darkness and ceases with sunrise. In the 1980s, the importance of melatonin in synchronizing the circadian rhythms in human beings was first discovered. A gradual decrease of melatonin levels in 11–15 year olds was found, with the assumption that melatonin depresses puberty and that during adolescence there is a decreased secretion of the hormone in order to allow appropriate sexual development [50]. Another change in adolescence is the 30–45-min delay in melatonin secretion, which in turn affects the sleep-wake rhythms and causes later sleep onset in adolescents than in children [5, 51].

In one study, Carskadon et al. [51] examined the circadian physiological changes (by way -of melatonin as a signal) that take place during adolescence. It was found that in the transition from 9th to 10th grade, the onset of melatonin secretion (Dim Light Melatonin Onset—DLMO) was extended by 30 min, even though school began 65 min earlier. Another study [52] compared the circadian rhythms of adolescents (mean age 16) and young adults (mean age 25) by examining their melatonin secretion and sleep-wake cycles in a naturalistic setting. A significant relationship was found between the melatonin secretion rhythm and sleep Chrono type (morning/evening) and natural sleeping habits. In other words, a later melatonin secretion rhythm manifests in evening sleep and late sleeping habits (late sleep onset and offset). However, no correlation was found between the level of sleepiness and the quality of sleep [4].

These findings point to similar circadian characteristics among adolescents and young adults. Like adults, adolescents react to sleep deprivation by increased physiological sleepiness due to a decrease in the amount and intensity of nocturnal deep sleep (Delta sleep), as well as by increased sleepiness during the short daytime sleep-wake cycles (MSLT), even when nocturnal sleep is not shortened. In other words, adolescents tend to easily fall asleep during the day when given the opportunity [53].

Eating Habits During Puberty: Psychopathological Perspective

Over the last five decades, there has been a dramatic cultural increase in the preference for thinness resulting in greater focus, among primarily adolescent and young adult women, on body shaper. Gradually, this is becoming true for males as well. In conjunction with the growing drive for thinness as the cultural ideal of beauty in modern Western societies, adolescents are increasingly prone to developing disordered eating and eating disorders [23, 54, 55]. Yet, in a paradoxical way, the more that thinness is emphasized as the model for happiness, the more the tendency to gain weight among children and adolescents increases. As a result, the diet industry continues to promote irregular and unbalanced eating habits and the use of destructive weight-regulation substances, such as laxatives, diuretics, enemas, fasting, and weight loss pills, along with compulsive exercise.

It has become increasingly clear that a large number of adolescents in non-clinical settings have abnormal eating attitudes and weight concerns that may require attention as the first signs of disordered eating pathology (sub-clinical eating disorders) [15, 23] and which if left untreated may develop into full-blown eating disorders [56]. Adolescents are likely to exhibit numerous behaviors designed to manage their weigh which may increase their risk for developing an eating disorder [15]. Research has shown that more than 50 % of students in the US exercise compulsively in order to lose weight, and 40 % restrict their eating [21]. Additionally, it was found that 80 % of adolescent girls with normal weight and height are not satisfied with their body shape and weight and wish to lose weight [20]. Studies in Israel assessing disordered eating attitudes and behaviors have shown that between 60–80 % of female adolescents are dissatisfied with their weight and shape, though the vast majority of these youngsters are of normal or even low weight [57]. Furthermore about 20 % presented maladaptive eating behavior, with 16–18-years-old girls having the highest disturbed eating-related patterns as compared to the other age groups [22, 58, 59] Recent research has found that about 30 % of adolescents met the criteria for disordered eating pathology [60] and almost 50 % of those who are diagnosed with EDNOS (Eating Disorders Not Otherwise Specified) may develop full-blown ED if left untreated. However it's important to note that disordered eating behaviors do not necessarily lead to the development of full-blown eating disorders later in life [61]. Full-blown of eating disorders are characterized by an obsessive preoccupation with food and body shape, coupled with unhealthy behaviors aimed at losing or maintaining weight in conjunction with low self-esteem and self-worth. The most common eating disorders are: Anorexia Nervosa (AN), Bulimia Nervosa (BN), Binge Eating Disorder (BED), and Eating Disorders Not Otherwise Specified (EDNOS) [55, 61].

Sleep Structure and Habits During Puberty: Psychopathological Perspective

Sleep psychopathology is associated with physiological and psychological aspects. Psychological factors that may influence sleep quality, found to be associated with mood disorders, anxiety disorders, and substances abuse while physiological factors are mainly demonstrated in circadian rhythm disorders (e.g., late sleep phase and/or unorganized biological clock) [62, 63]. Sleep disorders may be manifested in various psychiatric disorders, such as PTSD, affective disorders, and anxiety [33, 64]. Decreased and delayed sleep time may cause daytime fatigue and sleepiness, which in turn evokes stress and influences one's ability to function throughout the day [65].

Excessive daytime sleepiness is a very common complaint reported by approximately 25 % of adolescents, pointing to the need for more sleep time [66, 67]. Some adolescents consider sleep as an unimportant and ineffective activity in comparison to their academic and social activities. During weekdays, many adolescents get insufficient sleep because of their tendency to delay sleep and their early morning awakening for school [6]. Staying up late at night is also linked to a sense of autonomy and independence from their parents [67, 68]. Current research shows that most sleep problems will pass naturally over time. However, close to 15 % of teenagers and children do suffer from sleep disorders that require treatment [69]. Studies indicate a link between various sleeping problems and psychiatric comorbidity. Therefore, the treatment of sleep disorders is recommended in order to prevent the development of psychological problems in the future. Despite the lack of research on the connection between excessive sleepiness and stress among adolescents, there is a consensus among researchers that sleep deprivation adversely influences their daily functioning and increases the incidence of psychological and behavioral disorders [70, 71].

Only a few studies have examined the influence of sleep deprivation on cognitive performance in childhood and even less so on adolescents. The studies were conducted either in a laboratory or in a naturalistic environment at home, using an actigraph (objective measurement of the sleep-wake cycle) or subjective self-reports. The results have demonstrated the negative effects of adolescents' typical sleep patterns on their academic performance, cognitive and neurobehavioral functioning, emotional state, and risk-taking behavior [9, 62, 72]. It was found that [38] decreased sleep duration was associated with daytime fatigue and decreased cognitive performance in both children and adolescents. Moreover, simple cognitive functions, such as language skills, attentiveness, tasks and memory, became more difficult as a result of sleep deprivation. Students with low grades reported a bigger difference between school days and weekends in bedtime and wake-up time than did students with higher grades [36]. Other studies have shown similar results [73–75]. Fallone et al. [73] found that adolescents who slept less (i.e., 4 h) demonstrated daytime sleepiness, lack of attentiveness, restlessness, and slow reaction time in comparison to adolescents who slept through the night. A recent study indicated a significant relationship between longer sleep time (i.e., 8 h instead of six) and success on examinations [67, 76].

In addition it was found that [76] adolescents (between the ages of 12–18) slept an average of 8 ± 0.9 h on school days and 9.5 ± 1.65 h on the weekends. However when examined by age group, the group aged 12–13 slept 8.64 ± 0.8 h, whereas sleep time decreased to 7.8 ± 0.7 at age 16. Therefore, as adolescents get older, they sleep less during the week.

Recent studies conducted in Israel have examined the relationship between sleep duration and cognitive performance among adolescents [77]. One study assessing Israeli adolescents (mean age 14) found that the students went to bed on average at 23:15 ± 0:55 and slept on average 7.6 ± 1 h. The students were asked to go to sleep an hour earlier. Results indicated that the students extended their sleep time on average by 38 min per night and significantly improved their attentiveness and concentration in comparison to their prior performance [78]. In another recent study, a similar result was found when wake-up time was prolonged by delaying the start of the school day by an hour, which resulted in increased cognitive performance, attentiveness, and concentration [77].

Overall, the transition from childhood to adolescence is associated with delayed sleep onset and subsequent sleep deprivation which is known to effect mood behavior and cognitive performance. These changes are engendered by alterations in neuroendocrine function, as well as social and psychological factors.

Sleep-Wake Cycles in Adolescents with Eating Disorders

Nutritional factors found to play a role in the sleep disturbances seen in people with psychiatric disorders [79, 80]. Several studies have documented this relationship among adolescents as well whose sleep patterns are intimately tied to emotional regulation and mood disorders [7, 31, 81] In addition, decreased sleep has consistently been associated with dysregulated eating in children and adolescents [1, 82, 83] Other eating and food-related problems, may play an important role in the development or severity of some sleep disorders [84, 85] such as food allergy insomnia, nocturnal eating syndrome, eating disorders, and Klein Levin Syndrome and more. Adolescents with ED tend to complain about sleep disturbances [61, 86]. Studies examining sleep disorders among patients with ED have used polysomnography test, self-report questionnaires or home ambulatory monitoring (i.e., actigraph). The actigraph was used in several studies conducted in Israel with adolescent girls diagnosed with eating disorders so as to monitor the sleep-wake cycle in the subject's natural environment [87]. These studies have contributed a great deal to demonstrating the relationship between eating and sleep disorders.

With regard to **Bulimia Nervosa**, there is evidence that some patients with bulimia nervosa (BN) reported sleep disturbances [83, 88, 89]. Several studies using sleep electroencephalograms (EEG) in BN patients have yielded conflicting findings [86]. Few Studies [90–92] reported similar sleep patterns to those of patients with major depression, such as shortened REM latency. In contrast, others [80, 93, 94] did not find altered REM sleep patterns in Patients with BN, regardless of the coexistence of major depression. Other studies have shown that the sleep EEG of BN patients with normal weight is similar to that of healthy control subjects [95]. In contrast to the EEG sleep laboratory research, a study conducted in Israel [96] using actigraphic monitoring for the first time revealed significant differences in the sleep-wake patterns of patients with BN, who had sleep onset followed by sleep termination on an average of 1 h later, as compared to healthy control. These differences in sleep-wake patterns cannot be demonstrated under laboratory conditions, as subjects' sleep and wake-up times are predetermined. However, it is important to note that the Actigraph records only sleep or awake conditions without assessing sleep stages. This average 1-h difference, is probably not the result of sleep disturbances, such as insomnia or phase delay, but rather the result of binge eating behavior during the evening. Previous research has shown that most patients with BN have difficulty in controlling their eating behavior when they are alone in unstructured situations [85]. This usually occurs during the evening hours, as these individuals are frequently calorie-deprived during the day [97]. In contrast to the objective results, clinical observations have repeatedly shown that BN patients complain of sleep disturbances, such as difficulty falling asleep, mid-sleep awakenings, early awakenings, excessive daytime sleepiness, restlessness, and headaches after awakening. The same discrepancies between subjective complaints of sleep disturbances and EEG findings were frequently observed in studies on posttraumatic stress disorder (PTSD) [98]. PTSD and BN patients alike may have a perceptual deviation that characterizes the clinical picture of both pathologies. Complaints of sleepiness during the day may also be connected to the aftermath of the binge episode, including vomiting, fasting during the day, rigorous exercising, laxative usage, and diuretic intake. The remaining subjective sleep complaints may be explained by the clinical picture of binge-purge eating behavior, with anger, depression, interpersonal sensitivity, affective instability, aggressive impulse expression, opposition acting out, self-punishment, and irritability [96].

Clinicians should be aware of the discrepancies between the objective sleep patterns and the subjective perceptions of BN patients regarding their sleep efficiency before considering pharmaceutical intervention. They should treat the patients' subjective sleep complaints in light of their distorted body image problem. In addition, further research is needed to assess the relationship between sleep disorders and patters and evening binge episodes in patients with BN [31, 81, 99].

Binge Eating Disorders found to be associated with overweight and obesity. Over the past few decades the prevalence of obesity among children and adolescents has grown to epidemic proportion, portends an obesity-related medical conditions, including cardiovascular diseases, type 2 diabetes mellitus, degenerative joint diseases [100], and breathing disorders during sleep [101, 102]. Numerous studies have consistently demonstrated a strong association between obesity and sleep disruption or deprivation [1, 2, 26, 82, 83] Some previous studies have shown that obesity is the most significant risk factor for obstructive sleep apnea (OSA) [84, 103]. Several studies have shown that as many as 94 % of overweight children suffer from a sleep disturbances [104], mainly sleep disordered breathing (SDB) or sleep apnea [101, 105]. Chay et al. [63] found that 13.3 % of youngsters in Singapore whose weight was higher than 180 % of their ideal body weight suffered from SDB, as compared with 0.7 % of youngsters whose weight was less than 180 % of their ideal body weight. However, the currently available epidemiological data for SDB among adolescents are limited [106]. To our knowledge, most of the studies related to sleep disorders among the overweight young population have been conducted on children, and actigraphic evaluations have rarely been carried out among overweight adolescents.

One study was conducted in Israel [107] using actigraphic monitoring in three groups of adolescents: (1) overweight, (2) overweight with binge eating disorder (BED), and (3) an age-matched control group. The results revealed no significant differences in any of the parameters of the objective sleep-wake cycle, which was found to be within the normal range for all three groups. These findings are in contrast with those of a previous study, which demonstrated lower sleep efficiency and more wakefulness during sleep among an obese BED adult group, as compared with a normal weight control group [108]. Gupta et al. [109] found that sleep disturbances among adolescents were not directly related to obesity, but rather to physical activity level. Thus, the authors suggested that differences between overweight adolescents may be related to psychological wellbeing or by the amount of physical activity, and not necessarily by sleep disturbances or BMI [110]. In addition it may also be related the adolescents late sleep-wake patterns (sleep onset and wake up late) [38, 111]. Therefore, findings from research conducted in a sleep laboratory may not reflect actual sleep patterns. Support for this explanation can be found in observations on overweight adolescents and children suffering from binge eating disorder, whose quality of sleep is lower than that of their overweight peers without binge eating episodes [107].

In order to examine this assumption, further polysomnographic, psychiatric and psychological evaluations must be conducted. It remains difficult to diagnose binge eating episodes among adolescents according to the proposed criteria of BED in the DSM-IV [112, 113]. Therefore it is suggested to focus more on the loss of control over eating rather than on the number of binging episodes and the amount of food eaten throughout each episode, during the assessment phase.

With regards to **Anorexia Nervosa (AN)**, studies assessing sleep disorders in patients with AN have led to conflicting results, yet there is an evidence that some AN patients have sleep abnormalities [114, 115]. Patients with AN evaluated in laboratory were found to have a greater reduction in sleep, particularly slow-wave sleep and REM sleep [93], shorter REM latency [79], low overall sleep time, and low sleep efficiency as compared to controls [116, 117]. However, other studies did not find significant differences in sleep quality and quantity between AN and controls [118, 119]. Furthermore, one study using actigraphic monitoring in the subjects' natural environment revealed no significant differences in the objective sleep-wake patterns between AN and control [96]. The authors suggest that the malnutrition associated with AN necessitates energy conservation and therefore, preserving sleep may serve as a defense mechanism. It is possible that normal sleep serves as a compensatory mechanism in reaction to a protracted, severe illness or stressor. The body is prepared for a prolonged stress situation by maintaining normal sleep patterns and thereby enabling mental and physical coping with the situation. In addition it is suggested that patients with AN disengages from the constant sensation of hunger and deny it. It is possible that during such disengagement from hunger, this compensatory mechanism is executed in order to preserve the performance of various systems, among them the sleep-wake pattern. This explanation is partially supported by research examining the relationship between sleep disorders and weight loss [79] and malnutrition [120]. These findings clearly indicate that the sleep pattern of AN patients is significantly different from that of depressive patients.

On the other hand, contrary to the objective results, anecdotal observations suggest that adolescent girls with AN report significantly more subjective sleep disturbances than a healthy control group. These disturbances included difficulty falling asleep, mid-sleep awakenings, excessive daytime sleepiness, and restlessness. A possible explanation given by the researchers is that these discrepancies may be related to the confused manner in which individuals with AN experience their bodies as being overweight even though they are underweight. Such distortions in body image and weight perception might be expressed as other somatic physiological complaints. In light of the above findings, the authors suggested that therapists should treat the subjective complaints about sleep disturbances in a similar manner to their distorted body image. Further investigation is necessary before we can clearly state that sleep disturbances are not present in AN patients.

A different phenomenon termed **Klein Levin syndrome** (KLS) is a rare, but potentially severe and difficult to diagnose, disorder of excessive sleepiness that combines eating and sleeping problems in adolescents. KLS has an episodic appearance, which characterized by hyper somnolence (100 %), sometimes accompanied with binge eating behavior, hyperphagia, cognitive, mood, and behavioral changes, and sexual disinhibition. Each attack may last between several days (usually over 3) and several weeks but usually last around 5–10 days. Recurring every several month (medium 3.5) between one attack per month and one per year or even less than that. The onset is commonly during adolescence (around age 15), with a higher occurrence in males. The typical duration from the first attack to complete remission is about 8 years [121].

It has been reported to occur after trauma or viral infections, such as Epstein–Barr virus (EBV) or cytomegalovirus (CMV). However, it is commonly idiopathic [121], with unknown etiology and pathophysiology. Theories suggest that [121], probably more than one mechanism leading to this syndrome and the clinical characteristic may change with specific etiological factors. Attacks may be precipitated by febrile disease, strong emotions, or stress. It is an important feature that between attacks, affected individuals are typically completely asymptomatic and healthy, both physically and mentally. The attacks tends to decrease with age, and each episodes become shorter and it eventually remits spontaneously, yielding an excellent prognosis.

Conclusion

Adolescence is an age with many transitions and changes occurring in all areas, including in eating and sleeping habits. The combination of physiological and behavioral changes is likely to result in a vicious cycle of shorter sleep duration that leads to sleepiness and fatigue during the day; a decrease in mood; lower cognitive, behavioral, and social function; reduced energy; less interest in physical activity; lower calorie expenditure; and weight gain [122, 123] as well as increased consumption [9, 83]. As most of these changes are normative, it is therefore essential to separate them from pathological patterns and to identify risk factors for eating disorders, such as rapid weight loss, dieting behavior, body dissatisfaction, low self-esteem, mood fluctuation, social isolation, amenorrhea, compulsive exercise, and preoccupation with food, weight, and body shape.

Given the evidence presented here on the sleep-wake cycle in adolescents with AN, BN, BED, and NES, it appears that further research is needed in order to get a complete picture of the relation between eating and sleeping in different stages of adolescence. Future studies should consider such mediating factors as stress, personality type, mental status, coping mechanisms, peer pressure, family influence, parental supervision, and socio-cultural values.

Take home points

- Adolescence is an age with many transitions and changes occurring in all areas, including in eating and sleeping habits.
- In contrast to children, adolescents go to sleep much later and experience a significant delay in sleep onset, both during the week and even more so on the weekend.
- Sleep duration recommended for adolescents is between 8–9 h.
- The negative effects of adolescents' sleep deprivation are reflected on their academic performance, cognitive and neurobehavioral functioning, emotional state, and risk-taking behavior.
- Adolescents tend to the extreme in their eating behavior and food choices, often trying diverse types of diets.
- Although adolescents need a balanced diet in order to meet all of their developmental requirements, they often do not choose the appropriate food and instead consume high-calorie fast food while eating out with their friends.
- Adolescents are also inclined to avoid family meals and to skip breakfast.
- Adolescents are profoundly influenced by their peers and by the media, are keen on following the latest trends in nutrition and diet, and are subject to superstitions and myths about eating that have no connection to any proven nutritional quality.
- As most of these changes are normative, it is essential to separate them from pathological patterns and to identify risk factors for eating and sleeping disorders in adolescence.

References

1. Hart CN, Carskadon MA, Considine RV, Fava JL, Lawton J, Raynor HA, et al. Changes in children's sleep duration on food intake, weight, and leptin. Pediatrics. 2013;132(6): e1473–80.
2. Randler C, Haun J, Schaal S. Assessing the influence of sleep-wake variables on body mass index (BMI) in adolescents. Eur J Psychol. 2013;9(2):339–47.
3. Steinberg L. Adolescence. Boston, MA: McGraw-Hill, Inc; 1999.
4. Colrain IM, Baker FC. Changes in sleep as a function of adolescent development. Neuropsychol Rev. 2011;21(1):5–21.
5. Campbell IG, Grimm KJ, de Bie E, Feinberg I. Sex, puberty, and the timing of sleep EEG measured adolescent brain maturation. Proc Natl Acad Sci USA. 2012;109(15):5740–3.
6. Leger D, Beck F, Richard J, Godeau E. Total sleep time severely drops during adolescence. 2012.
7. Owens J. Adolescent Sleep Working Group, Committee on Adolescence. Insufficient sleep in adolescents and young adults: an update on causes and consequences. Pediatrics. 2014;134 (3):e921–32.
8. Sater E. Children eating from childhood to adulthood. Tel-Aviv: Zmora-Bitan; 1991.
9. Beebe DW. Cognitive, behavioral, and functional consequences of inadequate sleep in children and adolescents. Pediatr Clin North Am. 2011;58(3):649–65.
10. Carskadon MA. Sleep in adolescents: the perfect storm. Pediatr Clin North Am. 2011;58 (3):637–47.
11. Shochat T, Cohen-Zion M, Tzischinsky O. Functional consequences of inadequate sleep in adolescents: a systematic review. Sleep Med Rev. 2014;18(1):75–87.
12. Zuromski KL, Witte TK, Smith AR, Goodwin N, Bodell LP, Bartlett M, et al. Increased prevalence of vegetarianism among women with eating pathology. Eat Behav. 2015;19:24–7.
13. Beck C. Nourishing your daughter: help your child develop a healthy relationship with food and her body < br/> USA. New york, NY: Berkley Publishing group, A division of Penguim Putnam Inc; 2001.
14. Salvy S, De La Haye K, Bowker JC, Hermans RC. Influence of peers and friends on children's and adolescents' eating and activity behaviors. Physiol Behav. 2012;106(3): 369–78.
15. Snoek HM, Engels RC, van Strien T, Otten R. Emotional, external and restrained eating behaviour and BMI trajectories in adolescence. Appetite. 2013;67:81–7.
16. Lundgren JD, Allison KC, Crow S, O'Reardon JP, Berg KC, Galbraith J, et al. Prevalence of the night eating syndrome in a psychiatric population. Am J Psychiatry. 2014.
17. Meule A, Allison KC, Platte P. Emotional eating moderates the relationship of night eating with binge eating and body mass. Eur Eat Disord Rev. 2014;22(2):147–51.
18. Nolan LJ, Geliebter A. Night eating is associated with emotional and external eating in college students. Eat Behav. 2012;13(3):202–6.
19. Fairburn CG, Harrison PJ. Eat disorders. Lancet. 2003;361(9355):407–16.
20. Jones JM, Bennett S, Olmsted MP, Lawson ML, Rodin G. Disordered eating attitudes and behaviours in teenaged girls: a school-based study. CMAJ. 2001;165(5):547–52.
21. Kann L, Kinchen SA, Williams BI, Ross JG, Lowry R, Grunbaum JA, et al. Youth risk behavior surveillance–United States, 1999. MMWR CDC Surveill Summ. 2000;49(5):1–32.
22. Latzer Y, Witztum E, Stein D. Eating disorders and disordered eating in Israel: an updated review. Eur Eat Disord Rev. 2008;16(5):361–74.
23. Neumark-Sztainer D, Wall M, Larson NI, Eisenberg ME, Loth K. Dieting and disordered eating behaviors from adolescence to young adulthood: findings from a 10-year longitudinal study. J Am Diet Assoc. 2011;111(7):1004–11.
24. Adamo KB, Wilson S, Belanger K. Later bedtime is associated with greater daily energy intake and screen time in obese adolescents independent of sleep duration. The Complexity of Adolescent Obesity: Causes, Correlates, and Consequences 2014:37.

25. Beebe DW, Simon S, Summer S, Hemmer S, Strotman D, Dolan LM. Dietary intake following experimentally restricted sleep in adolescents. Sleep. 2013;36(6):827–34.
26. Garaulet M, Ortega F, Ruiz J, Rey-Lopez J, Beghin L, Manios Y, et al. Short sleep duration is associated with increased obesity markers in European adolescents: effect of physical activity and dietary habits. The HELENA study. Int J Obes. 2011;35(10):1308–17.
27. Kohler M, van den Heuvel C. Is there a clear link between overweight/obesity and sleep disordered breathing in children? Sleep Med Rev. 2008;12(5):347–61.
28. de Heredia FP, Garaulet M, Gómez-Martínez S, Díaz LE, Wärnberg J, Androutsos O, et al. Self-reported sleep duration, white blood cell counts and cytokine profiles in European adolescents: the HELENA study. Sleep Med. 2014;15(10):1251–8.
29. Dewald-Kaufmann JF, Oort FJ, Bögels SM, Meijer AM. Why sleep matters: differences in daytime functioning between adolescents with low and high chronic sleep reduction and short and long sleep durations. J Cogn Behav Psychotherapies. 2013;13(1a):171–82.
30. Dewald JF, Meijer AM, Oort FJ, Kerkhof GA, Bögels SM. The influence of sleep quality, sleep duration and sleepiness on school performance in children and adolescents: a meta-analytic review. Sleep Med Rev. 2010;14(3):179–89.
31. Roberts RE, Duong HT. The prospective association between sleep deprivation and depression among adolescents. Sleep. 2014;37(2):239–44.
32. Killgore W, Kahn-Greene E, Lipizzi E, Newman R, Kamimori G, Balkin T. Sleep deprivation reduces perceived emotional intelligence and constructive thinking skills. Sleep Med. 2008;9(5):517–26.
33. Gregory AM, Sadeh A. Sleep, emotional and behavioral difficulties in children and adolescents. Sleep Med Rev. 2012;16(2):129–36.
34. Sleep Patterns, Eating Habits and Electronic Media Exposure among Adolescents. 10th Conference of the Israeli Society of Sleep Research. 2009.
35. Carskadon MA. Patterns of sleep and sleepiness in adolescents. Pediatrician. 1990;17(1):5–12.
36. Hasler BP, Dahl RE, Holm SM, Jakubcak JL, Ryan ND, Silk JS, et al. Weekend–weekday advances in sleep timing are associated with altered reward-related brain function in healthy adolescents. Biol Psychol. 2012;91(3):334–41.
37. Wolfe P. Advice for the sleep-deprived. Educ Leadersh. 2005;23:39–40.
38. Wolfson AR, Carskadon MA. Sleep schedules and daytime functioning in adolescents. Child Dev. 1998;69(4):875–87.
39. Banks K. What a Research Says About Teenagers and Sleep. 2001 March, 2001;01.25:850.
40. Epstein R, Chillag N, Lavie P. Starting times of school: effects on daytime functioning of fifth-grade children in Israel. Sleep. 1998;21(3):250–6.
41. Andrade MM, Benedito-Silva AA, Menna-Barreto L. Correlations between morningness-eveningness character, sleep habits and temperature rhythm in adolescents. Braz J Med Biol Res. 1992;25(8):835–9.
42. Matricciani L, Olds T, Petkov J. In search of lost sleep: secular trends in the sleep time of school-aged children and adolescents. Sleep Med Rev. 2012;16(3):203–11.
43. Short MA, Gradisar M, Wright H, Lack LC, Dohnt H, Carskadon MA. Time for bed: parent-set bedtimes associated with improved sleep and daytime functioning in adolescents. Sleep. 2011;34(6):797–800.
44. Delaying school start time by one hour: effects on cognitive performance in adolescents; 2008.
45. Paksarian D, Rudolph KE, He J, Merikangas KR. School start time and adolescent sleep patterns: results from the US national comorbidity survey—adolescent supplement. Am J Public Health 2015(0):e1–e7.
46. O'Malley EB, O'Malley MB. School start time and its impact on learning and behaviour. Sleep. In: Ivanenko A, ed. and Psychiatric Disorders in Children and Adolescents New York, London: Informa healthcare; 2008.
47. Colrain IM. Sleep and the brain. Neuropsychol Rev. 2011;21(1):1–4.

48. Carskadon MA, Dement WC. The multiple sleep latency test: what does it measure? Sleep. 1982;5(Suppl 2):S67–72.
49. Borbely AA, Baumann F, Brandeis D, Strauch I, Lehmann D. Sleep deprivation: effect on sleep stages and EEG power density in man. Electroencephalogr Clin Neurophysiol. 1981;51 (5):483–95.
50. Crowley SJ, Acebo C, Carskadon MA. Human puberty: salivary melatonin profiles in constant conditions. Dev Psychobiol. 2012;54(4):468–73.
51. Carskadon MA, Wolfson AR, Acebo C, Tzischinsky O, Seifer R. Adolescent sleep patterns, circadian timing, and sleepiness at a transition to early school days. Sleep. 1998;21(8): 871–81.
52. Laberge L, Carrier J, Lesperance P, Lambert C, Vitaro F, Tremblay RE, et al. Sleep and circadian phase characteristics of adolescent and young adult males in a naturalistic summertime condition. Chronobiol Int. 2000;17(4):489–501.
53. Rosenthal L, Roehrs TA, Rosen A, Roth T. Level of sleepiness and total sleep time following various time in bed conditions. Sleep. 1993;16(3):226–32.
54. Smink FR, van Hoeken D, Hoek HW. Epidemiology of eating disorders: incidence, prevalence and mortality rates. Curr Psychiatry Rep. 2012;14(4):406–14.
55. Treasure J, Cladino AM, Zucke N. Eating disorders. Lancet. 2010;375:583–93.
56. Levine M, Smolak L. Toward a model of the developmental psychopathology of eating disorders: the example of early adolescence. The etiology of bulimia nervosa: The individual and familial context; 2013. p. 59–80.
57. Harel Y, Ellenbogen-Frankovits S, Molcho M, Abu-Ashas K, Habib J. Youth in Israel. Jerusalem, Israel: Brookdale Institute; 2002.
58. Greenberg L, Cwikel J, Mirsky J. Cultural correlates of eating attitudes: a comparison between native-born and immigrant university students in Israel. Int J Eat Disord. 2007;40 (1):51–8.
59. Latzer Y, Tzischinsky O. Weight concern, dieting and eating behaviors. A survey of Israeli high school girls. Int J Adolesc Med Health 2003 Oct–Dec;15(4):295–305.
60. Kaluski DN, Natamba BK, Goldsmith R, Shimony T, Berry EM. Determinants of disordered eating behaviors among Israeli adolescent girls. Eat Disord 2008 Mar-Apr;16(2):146–59.
61. Fairburn CG, Harrison PJ. Eating disorders. Lancet. 2003;361(9355):407–16.
62. Baum KT, Desai A, Field J, Miller LE, Rausch J, Beebe DW. Sleep restriction worsens mood and emotion regulation in adolescents. J Child Psychol Psychiatry. 2014;55(2):180–90.
63. Brand S, Gerber M, Kalak N, Kirov R, Lemola S, Clough PJ, et al. Adolescents with greater mental toughness show higher sleep efficiency, more deep sleep and fewer awakenings after sleep onset. J Adolesc Health. 2014;54(1):109–13.
64. American Psychiatric Association Committee on Nomenclature,and Statistics. Diagnostic and Statistical Manual of Mental Disorders (DSM–IV), 4th ed. Washington, DC: American Psychiatric Association; 1994.
65. Malone SK. Early to bed, early to rise?: an exploration of adolescent sleep hygiene practices. J Sch Nurs. 2011;27(5):348–54.
66. Fallone G, Owens JA, Deane J. Sleepiness in children and adolescents: clinical implications. Sleep Med Rev. 2002;6(4):287–306.
67. Morrison DN, McGee R, Stanton WR. Sleep problems in adolescence. J Am Acad Child Adolesc Psychiatry. 1992;31(1):94–9.
68. Fallone G, Seifer R, Acebo C, Carskadon MA. How well do school-aged children comply with imposed sleep schedules at home? Sleep. 2002;25(7):739–45.
69. Ford DE, Kamerow DB. Epidemiologic study of sleep disturbances and psychiatric disorders. An opportunity for prevention? JAMA. 1989;262(11):1479–84.
70. Harvey AG, Murray G, Chandler RA, Soehner A. Sleep disturbance as transdiagnostic: consideration of neurobiological mechanisms. Clin Psychol Rev. 2011;31(2):225–35.
71. Shanahan L, Copeland WE, Angold A, Bondy CL, Costello EJ. Sleep problems predict and are predicted by generalized anxiety/depression and oppositional defiant disorder. J Am Acad Child Adolesc Psychiatry. 2014;53(5):550–8.

72. Acebo C, Carskadon MA. Influence of irregular sleep patterns on waking behavior. In: Carskadon MA, ed. Adolescent Sleep Patterns: Biological, Social, and Psychological Influences New York: Cambridge University Press; 2002.
73. Fallone G, Acebo C, Arnedt JT, Seifer R, Carskadon MA. Effects of acute sleep restriction on behavior, sustained attention, and response inhibition in children. Percept Mot Skills. 2001;93(1):213–29.
74. Gozal D. Sleep-disordered breathing and school performance in children. Pediatrics. 1998;102(3 Pt 1):616–20.
75. Sadeh A, Acebo C. The role of actigraphy in sleep medicine. Sleep Med Rev. 2002;6 (2):113–24.
76. Loessl B, Valerius G, Kopasz M, Hornyak M, Riemann D, Voderholzer U. Are adolescents chronically sleep-deprived? An investigation of sleep habits of adolescents in the Southwest of Germany. Child Care Health Dev. 2008;34(5):549–56.
77. Tzchishinsky O, Shochat T, Lufi D. Reliability of the children's sleep habits questionnaire hebrew translation and cross cultural comparison of psychometric properties. Sleep Diagn Ther. 2008;3(3):30–4.
78. Gasol N, Tzischinsky O, Lufi D. The effects of sleep-wake cycle on the cognitive performance among adolescent. Researchers in the Emek Compilation of Articles Written by researchers at Max Stern Academic College of Emek yezreel; 2006.
79. Delvenne V, Kerkhofs M, Appelboom-Fondu J, Lucas F, Mendlewicz J. Sleep polygraphic variables in anorexia nervosa and depression: a comparative study in adolescents. J Affect Disord. 1992;25(3):167–72.
80. Lauer CJ, Krieg JC, Riemann D, Zulley J, Berger M. A polysomnographic study in young psychiatric inpatients: major depression, anorexia nervosa, bulimia nervosa. J Affect Disord. 1990;18(4):235–45.
81. Sarchiapone M, Mandelli L, Carli V, Iosue M, Wasserman C, Hadlaczky G, et al. Hours of sleep in adolescents and its association with anxiety, emotional concerns, and suicidal ideation. Sleep Med. 2014;15(2):248–54.
82. Burt J, Dube L, Thibault L, Gruber R. Sleep and eating in childhood: a potential behavioral mechanism underlying the relationship between poor sleep and obesity. Sleep Med. 2014;15 (1):71–5.
83. Lytle LA, Pasch KE, Farbakhsh K. The relationship between sleep and weight in a sample of adolescents. Obesity. 2011;19(2):324–31.
84. Association American Sleep Disorders. Thorpy MJ, Chairman, Rochester MN. International classification of sleep disorders: Diagnostic and coding manual, Diagnostic classification steering committee; 1990.
85. Harb A, Levandovski R, Oliveira C, Caumo W, Allison KC, Stunkard A, et al. Night eating patterns and chronotypes: a correlation with binge eating behaviors. Psychiatry Res. 2012;200(2):489–93.
86. Bos SC, Soares MJ, Marques M, Maia B, Pereira AT, Nogueira V, et al. Disordered eating behaviors and sleep disturbances. Eat Behav. 2013;14(2):192–8.
87. Tzischinsky O, Latzer Y. Sleep-wake cycle among adolescents who suffer from eating disorders: original Israeli research studies. Harefuah 2009 May; 148(5):322–8, 349.
88. Lombardo C, Battagliese G, Venezia C, Salvemini V. Persistence of poor sleep predicts the severity of the clinical condition after 6 months of standard treatment in patients with eating disorders. Eating Behav. 2015;18:16–9.
89. Trace SE, Thornton LM, Runfola CD, Lichtenstein P, Pedersen NL, Bulik CM. Sleep problems are associated with binge eating in women. Int J Eat Disord. 2012;45(5):695–703.
90. Katz JL, Kuperberg A, Pollack CP, Walsh BT, Zumoff B, Weiner H. Is there a relationship between eating disorder and affective disorder? New evidence from sleep recordings. Am J Psychiatry. 1984;141(6):753–9.
91. Neil JF, Merikangas JR, Foster FG, Merikangas KR, Spiker DG, Kupfer DJ. Waking and all-night sleep EEG's in anorexia nervosa. Clin Electroencephalogr. 1980;11(1):9–15.

92. Walsh BT, Goetz R, Roose SP, Fingeroth S, Glassman AH. EEG-monitored sleep in anorexia nervosa and bulimia. Biol Psychiatry. 1985;20(9):947–56.
93. Levy AB, Dixon KN, Schmidt H. Sleep architecture in anorexia nervosa and bulimia. Biol Psychiatry. 1988;23(1):99–101.
94. Hudson JL, Pope HG, Jonas JM, Stakes W, Grochocinski V, Lipinski JF, et al. Sleep EEG in bulimia. Biol Psychiat. 1987;22:820–8.
95. Levy AB, Dixon KN, Stern SL. How are depression and bulimia related? Am J Psychiatry. 1989;146(2):162–9.
96. Latzer Y, Tzischinsky O, Epstein R. Sleep-wake monitoring in women suffering from anorexia nervosa. Eat Disord 2001 Summer; 9(2):159–66.
97. Garner DM, Garfinkel PE. Handbook of psychotherapy for anorexia nervosa and bulimia. New York: Guilford Press; 1985.
98. Dagan Y, Lavie P, Bleich A. Elevated awakening thresholds in sleep stage 3–4 in war-related post-traumatic stress disorder. Biol Psychiatry. 1991;30(6):618–22.
99. Schmidt S, Randler C. Morningness-eveningness and eating disorders in a sample of adolescent girls. Journal of Individual Differences 2015.
100. Barlow SE, Dietz WH, Klish WJ, Trowbridge FL. Medical evaluation of overweight children and adolescents: reports from pediatricians, pediatric nurse practitioners, and registered dietitians. Pediatrics. 2002;110(1 Pt 2):222–8.
101. Redline S, Tishler PV, Schluchter M, Aylor J, Clark K, Graham G. Risk factors for sleep-disordered breathing in children. Associations with obesity, race, and respiratory problems. Am J Respir Crit Care Med 1999 May;159(5 Pt 1):1527–32.
102. Yuan H, Schwab RJ, Kim C, He J, Shults J, Bradford R, et al. Relationship between body fat distribution and upper airway dynamic function during sleep in adolescents. Sleep. 2013;36 (8):1199–207.
103. Sloan EP, Shapiro CM. Obstructive sleep apnea in a consecutive series of obese women. Int J Eat Disord. 1995;17(2):167–73.
104. Tzischinsky O, Latzer Y. Sleep-wake cycles in obese children with and without binge-eating episodes. J Paediatr Child Health. 2006;42(11):688–93.
105. Chay OM, Goh A, Abisheganaden J, Tang J, Lim WH, Chan YH, et al. Obstructive sleep apnea syndrome in obese Singapore children. Pediatr Pulmonol. 2000;29(4):284–90.
106. Amin R, Daniels S. Relationship between obesity and sleep-disordered breathing in children: is it a closed loop? J Pediatr. 2002;140(6):641–3.
107. Tzischinsky O, Latzer Y. Sleep-Wake cycles in obese adolescents with and without Binge Eating Episodes. Eur Eat Disord Rev. 2006;13:1–7.
108. Tzischinsky O, Latzer Y, Epstein R, Tov N. Sleep-wake cycles in women with binge eating disorder. Int J Eat Disord. 2000;27(1):43–8.
109. Gupta NK, Mueller WH, Chan W, Meininger JC. Is obesity associated with poor sleep quality in adolescents? Am J Hum Biol 2002 Nov-Dec;14(6):762–8.
110. Isnard P, Michel G, Frelut ML, Vila G, Falissard B, Naja W, et al. Binge eating and psychopathology in severely obese adolescents. Int J Eat Disord. 2003;34(2):235–43.
111. Golley RK, Maher C, Matricciani L, Olds T. Sleep duration or bedtime & quest; exploring the association between sleep timing behaviour, diet and BMI in children and adolescents. Int J Obes. 2013;37(4):546–51.
112. Ackard DM, Neumark-Sztainer D, Story M, Perry C. Over eating among adolescents: prevalence and associations with weight-related characteristics and psychological health. Pediatrics. 2003;111(1):67–74.
113. Morgan CM, Yanovski SZ, Nguyen TT, McDuffie J, Sebring NG, Jorge MR, et al. Loss of control over eating, adiposity, and psychopathology in overweight children. Int J Eat Disord. 2002;31(4):430–41.
114. Jauregui-Lobera I. Electroencephalography in eating disorders. Neuropsychiatr Dis Treat. 2012;8:1–11.

115. Vinai P, Ferri R, Anelli M, Ferini-Strambi L, Zucconi M, Oldani A, et al. New data on psychological traits and sleep profiles of patients affected by nocturnal eating. Sleep Med 2015.
116. Benca RM, Casper RC. Sleep in eating disorders. In: Kryger MH, Roth T, Dement WC, editors. Principles and practice of sleep medicine. 2nd ed. London: W.B. Saunders; 1994. p. 927–33.
117. Benca RM, Obermeyer WH, Thisted RA, Gillin JC. Sleep and psychiatric disorders. A meta-analysis. Arch Gen Psychiatry 1992 Aug;49(8):651–68; discussion 669–70.
118. Gertman-Israel D. Sleep and Dreaming in Anorexia Nervosa. Jerusalem, Israel: Hebrew University; 1998.
119. Lauer C, Zulley J, Krieg JC, Riemann D, Berger M. EEG sleep and the cholinergic REM induction test in anorexic and bulimic patients. Psychiatry Res. 1988;26(2):171–81.
120. Nobili L, Baglietto MG, De Carli F, Savoini M, Schiavi G, Zanotto E, et al. A quantified analysis of sleep electroencephalography in anorectic adolescents. Biol Psychiatry. 1999;45 (6):771–5.
121. Arnulf I, Lin L, Gadoth N, File J, Lecendreux M, Franco P, et al. Kleine-Levin syndrome: a systematic study of 108 patients. Ann Neurol. 2008;63(4):482–93.
122. Spiegel K, Leproult R, Van Cauter E. Impact of sleep debt on metabolic and endocrine function. Lancet. 1999;354(9188):1435–9.
123. Van Helder T, Symons JD, Radomski MW. Effects of sleep deprivation and exercise on glucose tolerance. Aviat Space Environ Med. 2003;4:487–92.

Chapter 3
Endocrinopathies of Eating Disorders

Nehama Zuckerman-Levin, Yael Latzer, Patricia E. Dunne and Ze'ev Hochberg

Abstract The rise of eating disorders (EDs) globally and increase in cases reported among children, underscore the urgent need for a clearer understanding of the medical consequences of these disorders. Medical abnormalities in EDs engage the endocrine system, gastrointestinal tract, adipose tissue and sympathetic nervous system. Patients with EDs demonstrate endocrine dysregulation, which involves the hypothalamic-pituitary-adrenal axis with hypercortisolemia, the Growth Hormone-Insulin-Like Growth Factor (GH-IGF) axis through its effect on growth and bone health, and the hypothalamic-pituitary-gonadal axis through delayed puberty or hypogonadotrophic hypogonadism and amenorrhea. In most cases of emaciated patients, as in cases of anorexia nervosa, these features are related to malnutrition, weight loss, and adaptation to starvation. However, in other cases, such as in bulimia nervosa, these abnormalities exist in patients with stable weight. Patients with EDs also evidence abnormalities of the hypothalamic-pituitary-thyroid axis as well as osmoregulation disturbances. Nutritional rehabilitation and weight gain remain the most effective options for restoring the endocrine complex, with overall ED treatment outcome enhanced by early diagnosis and a multidisciplinary treatment approach.

N. Zuckerman-Levin (✉) · Y. Latzer
Psychiatric Division, Eating Disorders Institute,
Rambam Medical Center, Haifa, Israel
e-mail: zuckerln@netvision.net.il

Y. Latzer
Faculty of Social Welfare and Health Sciences, University of Haifa, Haifa, Israel

P.E. Dunne
Department of Clinical & Counseling Psychology, Teachers College,
Columbia University, New York, NY, USA

N. Zuckerman-Levin · Z. Hochberg
Rappaport Faculty of Medicine and Research Institute,
Technion-Israel Institute of Technology, Haifa, Israel

Y. Latzer and D. Stein (eds.), *Bio-Psycho-Social Contributions to Understanding Eating Disorders*, DOI 10.1007/978-3-319-32742-6_3

Introduction

In the last few decades, eating disorders (EDs) have increased in prevalence in many parts of the world, primarily among adolescent females. However, the age range in which the disorders are manifesting has broadened to include both children [1] as well as women in mid-life and older [2]. These developments demand greater awareness and understanding of the serious medical complications and health consequences associated with EDs.

Among the multiple systems of the body adversely impacted by an ED is the endocrine system, which is reflected in patients with EDs through endocrine dysregulation. Initially, the clinical picture of ED was ascribed to pituitary failure, while later in the 1970s, focus shifted to the hypothalamus and higher brain centers. The clinical picture that emerged involves most of the hypothalamic- pituitary axes. The contemporary understanding of the weight control mechanism indicates that new players, including tissues, such as the brain, adipose tissue, the gastrointestinal tract, and the sympathetic nervous system, together with the endocrine system, contribute to the ED pathology. Hormones and peptides hailing from those respective body systems work together to regulate the processes of satiety and hunger, weight control and energy regulation.

Accordingly, endocrine dysregulation in anorexia nervosa (AN) includes malfunctioning of the hypothalamic-pituitary-adrenal (HPA) axis, resulting in hypercortisolemia; impairment of the Growth Hormone-Insulin-Like Growth factor (GH-IGF) axis—or GH Resistance—which has deleterious effects on growth and bone health; and complications of the hypothalamic-pituitary-gonadal (HPG) axis, such as delayed puberty or hypogonadotrophic hypogonadism and amenorrhea. Problems involving the hypothalamic-pituitary-thyroid axis (HPT) and osmoregulation disturbances are also common in patients with AN. Although the typical clinical features associated with this dysregulation are most conspicuous in the malnourished patient, these indicators may present in patients spanning the full spectrum of EDs, from the malnourished, underweight AN patient to stable or normal weight bulimic patient (BN). In cases of malnutrition, such as in AN, these endocrine alterations are related to weight loss and adaption to starvation.

This chapter will focus on changes in the endocrine system, as a cause or consequence of an ED. We will begin with a discussion of body weight, body composition and energy regulation, and then describe the growth hormone-related alterations in EDs. Next, we describe the dysfunction of the thyroid axis, the dysregulation of the adrenal function, and the changes in vasopressin (VP) and osmoregulation in patients with EDs. We provide an overview of the role of the hypothalamic-pituitary-gonadal axis and brief descriptions of the adipocytes and GIT-derived hormones and peptides affected by EDs. Lastly, we review the literature in light of its clinical implications, the long-term effects on quality of life and well-being, and identify areas for further research. The impact of EDs on bones will be discussed in a separate chapter (Chap. 5).

Body Weight, Body Composition and the Energy Regulation Process

Maintaining body weight homeostasis is a life-long process that is both intricate and tightly controlled. Physical sensations such as hunger and satiety, as well as energy expenditure, body composition, and bone mass, are regulated via a complex network of orexigenic and anorexigenic hormones, peripheral and central signals of hormones, and cytokines and peptides. In patients with EDs, this delicate regulatory milieu becomes imbalanced, though it remains unclear whether such abnormalities constitute a factor in the development of the disease, or result from starvation or changes in dietary habits.

Individuals with AN, including both adults and adolescents, have less body fat and lean body mass than their normal-weight counterparts. Compared to healthy controls, adolescents with AN can show up to a 50 % reduction in fat mass and a 40 % reduction in body fat percentage [3]. Changes in regional fat distribution patterns, including a diminished percentage of trunk fat and decreased trunk/extremity fat ratio, also occur in these adolescents [4], and to an even greater extent, in adults with AN [5]. In female adolescents, these changes may be reversed following weight gain during recovery, such that the regional fat distribution profile is restored to near normal levels. Yet in adult women, increases in percentage of trunk fat accompanying weight gain during recovery may potentially exceed that of healthy adults [5]. Interestingly, adolescent boys with AN do not show a decrease in their percentage of trunk fat owing to their low testosterone levels [6].

Growth Hormone-Insulin Like Growth Factor (GH-IGF) Changes

Some of the most harmful consequences of EDs are inflicted on the GH-IGF axis, the results of which may include decreased height velocity, impaired growth, disturbances in bone development, and metabolic changes. Muscle atrophy and bone loss can also occur. Such consequences could prove particularly harmful to younger patients who are still growing, thus the increasing prevalence of EDs in young children and adolescents in recent years is especially troublesome. Typically, patients with AN display high GH [7–9], with low total, free, and bioactive IGF1 [10–12]—a profile that reflects GH resistance, which is present in over 50 % of cases. The low levels of GHBP observed in AN suggest reduced GH-receptor activity [13, 14], which may in turn be related to metabolic adaptation to caloric deprivation and weight loss. Circulating IGFI levels, which are also low in patients with AN due to reduced synthesis by the liver, signify nutritional status and correlate positively with BMI [9, 10], and are nutritionally regulated [15].

Evidence suggests that elevated GH levels in patients with AN may reflect an increased frequency of GH pulses in AN [8, 9]. These pulses are then superimposed on increased tonic GH secretion, with no change demonstrated in GH half-life [8, 9]. Negative correlations have also been found between GH secretion and nutritional status markers such as BMI, fat mass, and Leptin. High GH levels may be attributable to low IGF-1, elevated levels of gastric Ghrelin [16], and reduced adipose tissue Leptin [9, 17]. Furthermore, high hypothalamic GHRH and low somatostatin levels [8, 18] also influence the GH profile in AN.

Results from GH provocative tests in AN [19] have revealed impaired GH response to L-dopa and apomorphine, normal response to GHRH stimulation [7], and attenuated response to insulin-induced hypoglycemia. Administration of TRH has been found to stimulate GH secretion in AN. However, weight restoration in patients with AN does not always normalize GH provocative tests [19]. In contrast with AN, GH levels and response to stimulation in individuals with BN typically fall within the normal range [20], though IGF1 levels may be lower than normal, as is the case in underweight patients.

Disturbances in the GH-IGF axis in AN usually resolve after weight gain and nutritional recovery [10, 21]. Catch-up growth will ensue following weight gain if epiphyseal fusion has not yet occurred, and preservation of height potential will be determined by the duration of the disease, IGF1 levels, and the delay in bone age [22]. Unfortunately, results from AN treatments aimed at normalizing the GH-IGF axis via administration of supraphysiological recombinant human GH to women with AN, did not successfully overcome GH resistance [23].

Dysfunction of the Thyroid Axis

AN is commonly associated with a clinical presentation that resembles 'euthyroid sick syndrome,' displaying typical changes in peripheral thyroid hormones [24, 25]. Consequently, results of thyroid function tests in patients with AN reveal normal to low-normal levels of TSH, normal or low T4 levels, and low levels of T3, while reverse T3 levels are elevated [26–30]. As in other conditions of euthyroid sick syndrome [28], patients with AN typically show deiodination of T4 to reverse T3 as opposed to active T3. Furthermore, in patients with AN, low TT3 is also associated with decreased thyroidal T3 secretion in response to endogenous TSH [29]. Total T3 levels correlate directly with measures of nutritional status in AN, including BMI, fat mass, insulin, glucose, IGF1, and Leptin. The secretion of TSH is usually normal in AN, however its response to stimulation with TRH is subnormal or shows delayed maximal response [31]. This result may indicate hypothalamic-pituitary-thyroid (HPT) dysfunction or a change in the set point for TRH regulation.

The clinical picture of thyroid axis dysfunction in AN resembles hypothyroidism, as it includes bradycardia, hypothermia, constipation, dry skin, and low basal metabolic rate. However, hypothyroidism is not in fact present; therefore there is no need for thyroid hormone replacement. Instead, the appearance of these signs and symptoms in AN reflect a state of starvation and chronic illness. Factors credited with generating this clinical picture include an adaptive reaction of the

HPT axis to starvation, a lack of energy resources, a low Basal Metabolic Rate (BMR), and a decrease in oxygen consumption and metabolic needs. This adaptation to starvation is part of a nitrogen-conserving reaction and is related to reduced resting energy expenditure [32].

Evidence from ultrasonography of the thyroid gland in AN cases reveals markedly reduced thyroid volume as compared with controls, which indicates thyroid atrophy [33]. This reduction in thyroid volume remains evident even after correcting for volumes predicted based on body weight and age. When weight restoration occurs late in the course of nutritional rehabilitation [28, 29, 32], the levels of reverse T3 decrease, while the levels of T3 increase. Mild symptoms of hyperthyroidism with excessive T3 have also been described in AN patients during the recovery phase [34].

Although patients with BN usually demonstrate normal thyroid function tests, some studies have reported that T3 has been in the low-normal range [35]. The administration of TRH to individuals with BN resulted in delayed maximal response of TSH [31].

Adrenal Function Dysregulation

Patients with AN demonstrate a unique pattern of the adrenal function axis, wherein plasma cortisol levels and urinary free cortisol levels are elevated [36–38]; cortisol production is normal [39] or slightly increased when referring to body size [40]; and pulse frequency is increased [38]. In addition, cortisol half-life is prolonged and metabolic clearance rate is decreased, with low urinary metabolites [39]. Some patients with AN lose their diurnal rhythm of cortisol [37, 41]. Hypercortisolism is frequently observed in malnourished anorexics, in normal weight bulimics, and in normal weight patients with functional hypothalamic amenorrhea as well as primary affective disorders [42–44].

In patients with AN, levels of plasma CRH are elevated and levels of ACTH are normal, while in the CSF, CRH is elevated and ACTH is low or low-normal [36, 45, 46]. Dynamic testing of the hypothalamic-pituitary-adrenal (HPA) axis demonstrates abnormal cortisol suppression by Dexamethazone in AN [40, 45], and BN [47, 48], with excessive cortisol and blunted ACTH response to CRH [36]. This dysregulation of the HPA axis points to impaired feedback at the hypothalamus or above, while feedback at the pituitary level is normally maintained. Normal peripheral ACTH [43, 45] and studies of glucocorticoid receptors rule out glucocorticoid resistance [49].

Although patients with AN have high levels of circulating cortisol, they lack a Cushingoid habitus due to the reduced availability of nutrients. However, they evidence a number of features that can be attributed to cortisol excess [50], including amenorrhea, osteopenia, skeletal muscle myopathy, mood disorders, and neurocognitive dysfunction. Importantly, high cortisol levels in AN patients predicts the redistribution of lean body mass such that extremity lean mass decreases

[51]. Following recovery and weight gain in AN, at which point trunk fat accumulation can be seen [52], cortisol production rate declines and dynamic testing improves [36, 53]. Still, subtle dysregulation of the HPA axis may persist after recovery [54]. Along these lines, it has been demonstrated that adrenal glucocorticoids and androgen precursor secretion are dissociated in AN, with hypercortisolemia and preservation of normal DHEA secretion [55]. Women with AN have low [56] or normal [55, 57] adrenal androgens DHEA and DHEAS.

Vasoperssin (VP) and Osmoregulation Changes

AN initiates changes in osmoregulation and water balance, which account for patients with AN exhibiting abnormal VP levels, in addition to low plasma sodium and osmolality, and normal potassium levels and acid-base balance [58]. Alterations in osmoregulation in AN cases are associated with increased levels of VP in the cerebrospinal fluid and were attributed to an intrinsic defect in the hypothalamic-posterior-pituitary axis [59]. Patients with AN may have a concentrating defect that is primarily of renal origin [60]. A water deprivation test demonstrated that most patients with AN have an impaired ability to concentrate urine [58], reflecting an inappropriate response to VP.

The Role of the Hypothalamic-Pituitary-Gonadal Axis in EDs

Findings from clinical studies show that the hypothalamic-pituitary-gonadal (HPG) axis in AN varies according to age and stage of puberty. As with any case of malnutrition, pre-pubertal girls or boys who develop an ED, particularly AN, will experience delayed puberty [3]. Meanwhile, a female who had already started puberty at the time of ED onset will experience breast atrophy, a reduction in the size of the uterus and ovaries with few or missing follicles, vaginal atrophy, and primary amenorrhea. Following menarche, secondary amenorrhea, oligomenorrhea or irregularity of menses will ensue in pubertal girls. Hypothalamic amenorrhea was one of the essential DSM-IV diagnostic criteria for AN, but this is no longer the case as it is not a diagnostic requirement in the DSM-5 [61]. Although weight loss typically precedes amenorrhea, some patients experience amenorrhea before weight loss, and others reach extremely low weight with intact reproductive function [62–64].

The hormonal profile of patients with AN is consistent with hypogonadotrophic hypogonadism, which is characterized by a lack of pulsatility, low amplitude and/or frequency of LH and FSH, reduced basal levels of gonadotropins, and a pre-pubertal pattern of LH secretion [65], with an immature response of gonadotropins to GnRH [66]. Levels of free estradiol are depleted on account of HPG dysfunction and decreased extragonadal sources of estrogens. Additionally, the metabolism of estradiol via 16-hydroxylation in AN cases is diminished, with preference given to the formation of 2-hydroxyestrone over estriol [67]. What's more, the loss of body fat can lead to hypoestrogenemia through a lack of adequate conversion of androgens to estrogens [68]. Although androgen deficiency [56, 57] in AN is mainly ovarian, it can be adrenal or of mixed origin. Patients with AN were reported to have low free and total testosterone levels [57, 69], which are associated with anxiety, depression, and eating-disordered thinking and behavior [70]. However, short-term, low-dose testosterone was shown to improve depressive symptoms, spatial cognition, and markers of bone turnover in women with AN [71].

Studies indicate that basal prolactin levels are normal in AN, while TRH-stimulated prolactin demonstrates a delayed peak response, with normal levels [19]. Like their female counterparts, males with AN are also described as having low gonadotropins, a pre-pubertal pattern of LH secretion and low testosterone, though hypogonadism in males has not been as well characterized [72, 73]. Unfortunately, as of yet no studies examining the effect of androgen treatment in males with AN have been conducted.

The degree of HPG dysregulation in AN is contingent on several factors, including fat mass [74], Leptin and Ghrelin levels, psychological comorbidity, level of physical activity [75, 76] and BMI, which are required for normal HPG function [63, 68, 77]. That said, women with a higher proportion of body fat maintain menses despite weight reduction [64].

After gaining 90 % of ideal body weight, 86 % of patients with AN will resume normal menses within 6 months, whereas up to 32 % of patients with AN remain amenorrheic after 1 year despite weight recovery and return of normal secretory patterns of gonadotropins [77]. Girls with AN who fail to resume menses subsequent to weight gain should be evaluated for the lean form of polycystic ovary syndrome (PCOS).

In terms of reproductive capabilities, women with a history of AN have a higher incidence of miscarriages and Cesarean deliveries. Additionally, they are more likely to have premature delivery and children that are born small for their gestational age [78]. Hormonal dysfunction, menstrual disturbances, and infertility are also described in patients with BN with normal weight but not nearly as often as in cases of AN [79]. Such patients with BN evidence low LH and FSH amplitude and frequency [80, 81].

Adipocytes and GIT—Derived Hormones and Peptides

Insulin. Low glucose levels are common in AN. Patients with AN exhibit low body weight and low fat mass which are associated with lower levels of fasting insulin and glucose than those observed in normal-weight adolescent girls. In addition, measures of insulin resistance, such as HOMA-IR, are markedly reduced in AN, and insulin secretion in response to glucose challenge is below normal [38, 82, 83].

When the body is in a state of severe under-nutrition such as in AN, increased GH and cortisol levels may act as an adaptive mechanism to maintain euglycemia.

Adiponectin, an adipocytokine, mediates insulin sensitivity and resistance through its effects on PPAR-γ. Adiponectin levels in patients with AN have been reported to range from elevated to unchanged or low [82, 84, 85]. There is some indication that high adiponectin levels in AN may contribute to low BMD by increasing osteoclast activity. Adiponectin is an inverse predictor of bone density in adolescents with AN [82]. Weight recovery is associated with decreased adiponectin levels in AN, which reflects a pattern similar to controls who undergo improved insulin sensitivity [85].

Leptin is a fat-derived anorexigenic hormone, which acts through the induction of POMC into the hypothalamus [86] and the inhibition of NPY secretion [87]. In AN, peripheral levels of Leptin decline as a result of lower basal and pulsatile secretion [17], and possibly, because of deviations from the circadian secretion rhythm [88]. Low levels of Leptin reflect decreased fat mass and correspond to other measures of nutrition like BMI and IGF1. The Leptin deficiency observed in AN is thought to play a role in hypothalamic-pituitary-ovarian dysfunction, thus the resumption of menses is associated with an increase in Leptin levels [17, 73]. Unlike girls with AN, boys with AN do not evidence Leptin deficiency, despite having lower fat mass than normal-weight boys [6]. Leptin has central and peripheral, anabolic, and negative effects on bone [89], and Leptin deficiency is associated with low bone mass [90]. Evidence suggests that Leptin levels surge higher than normal following weight gain [91], though it appears that levels eventually normalize so long as recovery is maintained long-term [92].

Peptide YY^{3-36} (PYY) is a gut-derived anorexigenic hormone secreted following food consumption. It induces satiety by binding to the Y2 receptor of NPY, and inhibiting secretion of NPY and Agouti-Related Protein (AgRP) in the hypothalamus. Both boys [6] and girls [93, 94] with AN exhibit high PYY levels. Unlike many other hormones and peptides, PPY levels do not normalize following weight gain, suggesting that PYY may potentially play a role in mediating susceptibility to this disease [93, 94]. In addition, high PYY levels in AN may also contribute to bone loss, as evidenced by an association between PYY and low levels of bone turnover markers [93]. In adults with AN, high PYY predicts lower bone density [95].

Ghrelin plays a key role in signaling hunger and in activating the GH axis, as well as cortisol secretion. Ghrelin is an orexigenic gastric peptide hormone that induces the secretion of NPY and AgRP in the brain [96]. Patients with AN show elevated Ghrelin levels [16, 97] as compared to lean, healthy individuals. Furthermore, they exhibit less sensitivity to Ghrelin in terms of GH response and appetite than healthy controls [98]. These findings suggest that body composition does not exclusively control the level of Ghrelin [96]. Rather, a rise in Ghrelin may also stem from increased secretory burst amplitude and frequency [16, 98, 99]. As patients with AN gain weight, Ghrelin levels decrease [16].

Conclusions

Collectively, this chapter demonstrates that EDs are associated with multiple endocrine dysfunctions. These abnormalities may reflect the body's physiological adaptation to starvation, or may be evidence of long-term complications associated with EDs. Although the state of starvation induced by an ED is not permanent, some of the endocrine complications it engenders can have lasting effects. The deleterious effects of EDs on the GH-IGF and HPG axis in children, adolescents, and young adults, have the potential to adversely impact growth, body composition, and the onset and progression of puberty. Moreover, they may leave an enduring imprint, on an individual's Quality Of Life and well-being.

Along these lines, weight gain and the resumption of menses are important indicators of recovery in AN. In light of the fact that the vast majority of individuals develop an ED during a crucial developmental stage, weight gain should initially be the primary goal. Thus, nutritional rehabilitation and weight gain play a major role in restoring the endocrine complex and enable subsequent psychological interventions. Consequently, early diagnosis is important in order to prevent permanent endocrine damage in children and adolescents. It is imperative then that primary care physicians and gynecologists are able to identify 'red flag' symptoms of EDs in patients like amennorhea, delayed puberty, or low BMI for age, and differentiate them from other etiologies. Early multidisciplinary treatment [100] has been shown to lead to favorable prognosis, particularly in young patients [101]. In summary, this chapter draws attention to the crucial role that pediatricians with a specialization in endocrinology play in the diagnosis and treatment of EDs and the importance of their inclusion in the multidisciplinary treatment team.

In line with these clinical implications, further research investigating the complex relations between neuroendocrine, gastrointestinal, and fat tissue factors is needed. While current research continues to investigate the etiology of EDs, as well as their treatment, future research calls for a close collaboration between endocrinologists and clinical practitioners.

Take home points

- The clinical features of patients across the spectrum of EDs are hormonal in nature.
- The endocrinological dysfunction in EDs may be due to adaptation to starvation or because of other long-term EDs related complications.
- Imbalance in Growth Hormone–Insulin-Like Growth Factor (GH-IGF) and the hypothalamic-pituitary-gonadal (HPG) axis have a crucial impact on children, adolescents and young adults due to their developmental stage, by influencing growth, body composition, and puberty.
- These endocrinological complications may have a long-term impact on quality of life and well-being, and are important indicators of recovery from AN.
- Symptoms associated with endocrinological imbalance such as amenorrhea and delayed puberty may facilitate the early detection of an ED. Caregivers should

therefore bear in mind the possibility of an ED in any adolescent presenting with these symptoms.

- Nutritional rehabilitation and weight gain calculated according to height potential rather than current height, remain the most effective interventions for ED-related endocrine complexities.

References

1. Hoek HW. Incidence, prevalence and mortality of anorexia nervosa and other eating disorders. Curr Opin Psychiatry. 2006;19:389–94.
2. Ackard DM, Richter S, Frisch MJ, Mangham D, Cronemeyer CL. Eating disorder treatment among women forty and older: increases in prevalence over time and comparisons to young adult patients. J Psychosom Res. 2013;74:175–8.
3. Misra M, Aggarwal A, Miller KK, Almazan C, Worley M, Soyka LA, et al. Effects of anorexia nervosa on clinical, hematologic, biochemical, and bone density parameters in community-dwelling adolescent girls. Pediatrics. 2004;114:1574–83.
4. Misra M, Soyka LA, Miller KK, Grinspoon S, Levitsky LL, Klibanski A. Regional body composition in adolescents with anorexia nervosa and changes with weight recovery. Am J Clin Nutr. 2003;77:1361–7.
5. Grinspoon S, Thomas L, Miller K, Pitts S, Herzog D, Klibanski A. Changes in regional fat redistribution and the effects of estrogen during spontaneous weight gain in women with anorexia nervosa. Am J Clin Nutr. 2001;73:865–9.
6. Misra M, Katzman DK, Cord J, Manning SJ, Mickley D, Herzog DB, et al. Percentage extremity fat, but not percentage trunk fat, is lower in adolescent boys with anorexia nervosa than in healthy adolescents. Am J Clin Nutr. 2008;88:1478–84.
7. Scacchi M, Pincelli AI, Caumo A, Tomasi P, Delitala G, Baldi G, Cavagnini F. Spontaneous nocturnal growth hormone secretion in anorexia nervosa. J Clin Endocrinol Metab. 1997;82:3225–9.
8. Stoving RK, Veldhuis JD, Flyvbjerg A, Vinten J, Hangaard J, Koldkjaer OG, et al. Jointly amplified basal and pulsatile growth hormone (GH) secretion and increased process irregularity in women with anorexia nervosa: indirect evidence for disruption of feedback regulation within the GH-insulin-like growth factor I axis. J Clin Endocrinol Metab. 1999;84:2056–63.
9. Misra M, Miller KK, Bjornson J, Hackman A, Aggarwal A, Chung J, et al. Alterations in growth hormone secretory dynamics in adolescent girls with anorexia nervosa and effects on bone metabolism. J Clin Endocrinol Metab. 2003;88:5615–23.
10. Argente J, Caballo N, Barrios V, Munoz MT, Pozo J, Chowen JA, et al. Multiple endocrine abnormalities of the growth hormone and insulin-like growth factor axis in patients with anorexia nervosa: effect of short- and long-term weight recuperation. J Clin Endocrinol Metab. 1997;82:2084–92.
11. Stoving RK, Flyvbjerg A, Frystyk J, Fisker S, Hangaard J, Hansen-Nord M, Hagen C. Low serum levels of free and total insulin-like growth factor I (IGF-I) in patients with anorexia nervosa are not associated with increased IGF-binding protein-3 proteolysis. J Clin Endocrinol Metab. 1999;84:1346–50.
12. Stoving RK, Chen JW, Glintborg D, Brixen K, Flyvbjerg A, Horder K, Frystyk J. Bioactive insulin-like growth factor (IGF) I and IGF-binding protein-1 in anorexia nervosa. J Clin Endocrinol Metab. 2007;92:2323–9.
13. Hochberg Z, Hertz P, Colin V, Ish-Shalom S, Yeshurun D, Youdim MB, Amit T. The distal axis of growth hormone (GH) in nutritional disorders: GH-binding protein, insulin-like

growth factor-I (IGF-I), and IGF-I receptors in obesity and anorexia nervosa. Metabolism. 1992;41:106–12.
14. Counts DR, Gwirtsman H, Carlsson LM, Lesem M, Cutler GB Jr. The effect of anorexia nervosa and refeeding on growth hormone-binding protein, the insulin-like growth factors (IGFs), and the IGF-binding proteins. J Clin Endocrinol Metab. 1992;75:762–7.
15. Thissen JP, Ketelslegers JM, Underwood LE. Nutritional regulation of the insulin-like growth factors. Endocr Rev. 1994;15:80–101.
16. Misra M, Miller KK, Kuo K, Griffin K, Stewart V, Hunter E, et al. Secretory dynamics of ghrelin in adolescent girls with anorexia nervosa and healthy adolescents. Am J Physiol Endocrinol Metab. 2005;289:e347–56.
17. Misra M, Miller KK, Kuo K, Griffin K, Stewart V, Hunter E, et al. Secretory dynamics of leptin in adolescent girls with anorexia nervosa and healthy adolescents. Am J Physiol Endocrinol Metab. 2005;289:e373–81.
18. Stoving RK, Andersen M, Flyvbjerg A, Frystyk J, Hangaard J, Vinten J, et al. Indirect evidence for decreased hypothalamic somatostatinergic tone in anorexia nervosa. Clin Endocrinol (Oxf). 2002;56:391–6.
19. Newman MM, Halmi KA. The endocrinology of anorexia nervosa and bulimia nervosa. Endocrinol Metab Clin North Am. 1988;17:195–212.
20. Kiriike N, Nishiwaki S, Izumiya Y, Maeda Y, Kawakita Y. Thyrotropin, prolactin, and growth hormone responses to thyrotropin-releasing hormone in anorexia nervosa and bulimia. Biol Psychiatry. 1987;22:167–76.
21. Golden NH, Kreitzer P, Jacobson MS, Chasalow FI, Schebendach J, Freedman SM, Shenker IR. Disturbances in growth hormone secretion and action in adolescents with anorexia nervosa. J Pediatr. 1994;125:655–60.
22. Prabhakaran R, Misra M, Miller KK, Kruczek K, Sundaralingam S, Herzog DB, et al. Determinants of height in adolescent girls with anorexia nervosa. Pediatrics. 2008;121: e1517–23.
23. Fazeli PK, Lawson EA, Prabhakaran R, Miller KK, Donoho DA, Clemmons DR, et al. Effects of recombinant human growth hormone in anorexia nervosa: a randomized, placebo-controlled study. J Clin Endocrinol Metab. 2010;95:4889–97.
24. Cavalieri RR. The effects of nonthyroid disease and drugs on thyroid function tests. Med Clin North Am. 1991;75:27–39.
25. Chopra IJ. Clinical review 86: Euthyroid sick syndrome: is it a misnomer? J Clin Endocrinol Metab. 1997;82:329–34.
26. Moshang T, Parks JS, Baker L, Vaidya V, Utiger RD, Bongiovanni AM, Snyder PJ. Low serum triiodothyronine in patients with anorexia nervosa. J Clin Endocrinol Metab. 1975;40:470–3.
27. Croxson MS, Ibbertson HK. Low serum triiodothyronine (T3) and hypothyroidism in anorexia nervosa. J Clin Endocrinol Metab. 1977;44:167–74.
28. Leslie RD, Isaacs AJ, Gomez J, Raggatt PR, Bayliss R. Hypothalamo-pituitary-thyroid function in anorexia nervosa: influence of weight gain. Br Med J. 1978;2:526–8.
29. Kiyohara K, Tamai H, Takaichi Y, Nakagawa T, Kumagai LF. Decreased thyroidal triiodothyronine secretion in patients with anorexia nervosa: influence of weight recovery. Am J Clin Nutr. 1989;50:767–72.
30. Kvetny J. Thyroxine binding and cellular metabolism of thyroxine in mononuclear blood cells from patients with anorexia nervosa. J Endocrinol. 1983;98:343–50.
31. Norris PD, O'Malley BP, Palmer RL. The TRH test in bulimia and anorexia nervosa: a controlled study. J Psychiatr Res. 1985;19:215–9.
32. Onur S, Haas V, Bosy-Westphal A, Hauer M, Paul T, Nutzinger D, et al. L-tri-iodothyronine is a major determinant of resting energy expenditure in underweight patients with anorexia nervosa and during weight gain. Eur J Endocrinol. 2005;152:179–84.
33. Stoving RK, Bennedbaek FN, Hegedus L, Hagen C. Evidence of diffuse atrophy of the thyroid gland in patients with anorexia nervosa. Int J Eat Disord. 2001;29:230–5.

34. Moore R, Mills IH. Serum T3 and T4 levels in patients with anorexia nervosa showing transient hyperthyroidism during weight gain. Clin Endocrinol (Oxf). 1979;10:443–9.
35. Spalter AR, Gwirtsman HE, Demitrack MA, Gold PW. Thyroid function in bulimia nervosa. Biol Psychiatry. 1993;33:408–14.
36. Gold PW, Gwirtsman H, Avgerinos PC, Nieman LK, Gallucci WT, Kaye W, et al. Abnormal hypothalamic-pituitary-adrenal function in anorexia nervosa. Pathophysiologic mechanisms in underweight and weight-corrected patients. N Engl J Med. 1986;314:1335–42.
37. Putignano P, Dubini A, Toja P, Invitti C, Bonfanti S, Redaelli G, et al. Salivary cortisol measurement in normal-weight, obese and anorexic women: comparison with plasma cortisol. Eur J Endocrinol. 2001;145:165–71.
38. Misra M, Miller KK, Almazan C, Ramaswamy K, Lapcharoensap W, Worley M, et al. Alterations in cortisol secretory dynamics in adolescent girls with anorexia nervosa and effects on bone metabolism. J Clin Endocrinol Metab. 2004;89:4972–80.
39. Boyar RM, Hellman LD, Roffwarg H, Katz J, Zumoff B, O'Connor J, et al. Cortisol secretion and metabolism in anorexia nervosa. N Engl J Med. 1977;296:190–3.
40. Walsh BT, Katz JL, Levin J, Kream J, Fukushima DK, Hellman LD, et al. Adrenal activity in anorexia nervosa. Psychosom Med. 1978;40:499–506.
41. dos Santos E, dos Santos JE, Ribeiro RP, Rosa ESAC, Moreira AC, Silva de Sa MF. Absence of circadian salivary cortisol rhythm in women with anorexia nervosa. J Pediatr Adolesc Gynecol 2007;20:13-8
42. Mortola JF, Rasmussen DD, Yen SS. Alterations of the adrenocorticotropin-cortisol axis in normal weight bulimic women: evidence for a central mechanism. J Clin Endocrinol Metab. 1989;68:517–22.
43. Licinio J, Wong ML, Gold PW. The hypothalamic-pituitary-adrenal axis in anorexia nervosa. Psychiatry Res. 1996;62:75–83.
44. Lo Sauro C, Ravaldi C, Cabras PL, Faravelli C, Ricca V. Stress, hypothalamic-pituitary-adrenal axis and eating disorders. Neuropsychobiology 2008;57:95-115.
45. Gwirtsman HE, Kaye WH, George DT, Jimerson DC, Ebert MH, Gold PW. Central and peripheral ACTH and cortisol levels in anorexia nervosa and bulimia. Arch Gen Psychiatry. 1989;46:61–9.
46. Kaye WH, Gwirtsman HE, George DT, Ebert MH, Jimerson DC, Tomai TP, et al. Elevated cerebrospinal fluid levels of immunoreactive corticotropin-releasing hormone in anorexia nervosa: relation to state of nutrition, adrenal function, and intensity of depression. J Clin Endocrinol Metab. 1987;64:203–8.
47. Hughes PL, Wells LA, Cunningham CJ. The dexamethasone suppression test in bulimia before and after successful treatment with desipramine. J Clin Psychiatry. 1986;47:515–7.
48. Hudson JI, Pope HG Jr, Jonas JM, Laffer PS, Hudson MS, Melby JC. Hypothalamic-pituitary-adrenal-axis hyperactivity in bulimia. Psychiatry Res. 1983;8:111–7.
49. Invitti C, Redaelli G, Baldi G, Cavagnini F. Glucocorticoid receptors in anorexia nervosa and Cushing's disease. Biol Psychiatry. 1999;45:1467–71.
50. McLoughlin DM, Wassif WS, Morton J, Spargo E, Peters TJ, Russell GF. Metabolic abnormalities associated with skeletal myopathy in severe anorexia nervosa. Nutrition. 2000;16:192–6.
51. Misra M, Miller KK, Almazan C, Worley M, Herzog DB, Klibanski A. Hormonal determinants of regional body composition in adolescent girls with anorexia nervosa and controls. J Clin Endocrinol Metab. 2005;90:2580–7.
52. Walsh BT, Katz JL, Levin J, Kream J, Fukushima DK, Weiner H, Zumoff B. The production rate of cortisol declines during recovery from anorexia nervosa. J Clin Endocrinol Metab. 1981;53:203–5.
53. Mayer L, Walsh BT, Pierson RN Jr, Heymsfield SB, Gallagher D, Wang J, et al. Body fat redistribution after weight gain in women with anorexia nervosa. Am J Clin Nutr. 2005;81:1286–91.

54. Estour B, Pugeat M, Lang F, Lejeune H, Broutin F, Pellet J, et al. Rapid escape of cortisol from suppression in response to i.v. dexamethasone in anorexia nervosa. Clin Endocrinol (Oxf). 1990;33:45–52.
55. Lawson EA, Misra M, Meenaghan E, Rosenblum L, Donoho DA, Herzog D, et al. Adrenal glucocorticoid and androgen precursor dissociation in anorexia nervosa. J Clin Endocrinol Metab. 2009;94:1367–71.
56. Gordon CM, Grace E, Emans SJ, Feldman HA, Goodman E, Becker KA, et al. Effects of oral dehydroepiandrosterone on bone density in young women with anorexia nervosa: a randomized trial. J Clin Endocrinol Metab. 2002;87:4935–41.
57. Miller KK, Lawson EA, Mathur V, Wexler TL, Meenaghan E, Misra M, et al. Androgens in women with anorexia nervosa and normal-weight women with hypothalamic amenorrhea. J Clin Endocrinol Metab. 2007;92:1334–9.
58. Evrard F, da Cunha MP, Lambert M, Devuyst O. Impaired osmoregulation in anorexia nervosa: a case-control study. Nephrol Dial Transplant. 2004;19:3034–9.
59. Gold PW, Kaye W, Robertson GL, Ebert M. Abnormalities in plasma and cerebrospinal-fluid arginine vasopressin in patients with anorexia nervosa. N Engl J Med. 1983;308:1117–23.
60. Aperia A, Broberger O, Fohlin L. Renal function in anorexia nervosa. Acta Paediatr Scand. 1978;67:219–24.
61. American Psychiatric Association. Diagnostic and statistical manual of mental disorders. 5th ed. Arlington: APA; 2013. p. 5–25.
62. Crisp AH, Stonehill E. Relation between aspects of nutritional disturbance and menstrual activity in primary anorexia nervosa. Br Med J. 1971;3:149–51.
63. Golden NH, Shenker IR. Amenorrhea in anorexia nervosa: etiology and implications. Adolesc Med. 1992;3:503–18.
64. Miller KK, Grinspoon S, Gleysteen S, Grieco KA, Ciampa J, Breu J, et al. Preservation of neuroendocrine control of reproductive function despite severe undernutrition. J Clin Endocrinol Metab. 2004;89:4434–8.
65. Boyar RM, Katz J, Finkelstein JW, Kapen S, Weiner H, Weitzman ED, Hellman L. Anorexia nervosa. Immaturity of the 24-hour luteinizing hormone secretory pattern. N Engl J Med. 1974;291:861–5.
66. Roth JC, Kelch RP, Kaplan SL, Grumbach MM. FSH and LH response to luteinizing hormone-releasing factor in prepubertal and pubertal children, adult males and patients with hypogonadotropic and hypertropic hypogonadism. J Clin Endocrinol Metab. 1972;35:926–30.
67. Frisch RE, McArthur JW. Menstrual cycles: fatness as a determinant of minimum weight for height necessary for their maintenance or onset. Science. 1974;185:949–51.
68. Fishman J, Boyar RM, Hellman L. Influence of body weight on estradiol metabolism in young women. J Clin Endocrinol Metab. 1975;41:989–91.
69. Gordon CM, Goodman E, Emans SJ, Grace E, Becker KA, Rosen CJ, et al. Physiologic regulators of bone turnover in young women with anorexia nervosa. J Pediatr. 2002;141:64–70.
70. Miller KK, Wexler TL, Zha AM, Lawson EA, Meenaghan EM, Misra M, et al. Androgen deficiency: association with increased anxiety and depression symptom severity in anorexia nervosa. J Clin Psychiatry. 2007;68:959–65.
71. Miller KK, Grieco KA, Klibanski A. Testosterone administration in women with anorexia nervosa. J Clin Endocrinol Metab. 2005;90:1428–33.
72. Rigotti NA, Neer RM, Jameson L. Osteopenia and bone fractures in a man with anorexia nervosa and hypogonadism. Jama. 1986;256:385–8.
73. Misra M, Katzman DK, Cord J, Manning SJ, Mendes N, Herzog DB, et al. Bone metabolism in adolescent boys with anorexia nervosa. J Clin Endocrinol Metab. 2008;93:3029–36.
74. Misra M, Prabhakaran R, Miller KK, Tsai P, Lin A, Lee N, et al. Role of cortisol in menstrual recovery in adolescent girls with anorexia nervosa. Pediatr Res. 2006;59:598–603.
75. Gendall KA, Joyce PR, Carter FA, McIntosh VV, Jordan J, Bulik CM. The psychobiology and diagnostic significance of amenorrhea in patients with anorexia nervosa. Fertil Steril. 2006;85:1531–5.

76. Jacoangeli F, Masala S, Staar Mezzasalma F, Fiori R, Martinetti A, Ficoneri C, et al. Amenorrhea after weight recover in anorexia nervosa: role of body composition and endocrine abnormalities. Eat Weight Disord. 2006;11:e20–6.
77. Golden NH, Jacobson MS, Schebendach J, Solanto MV, Hertz SM, Shenker IR. Resumption of menses in anorexia nervosa. Arch Pediatr Adolesc Med. 1997;151:16–21.
78. Bulik CM, Sullivan PF, Fear JL, Pickering A, Dawn A, McCullin M. Fertility and reproduction in women with anorexia nervosa: a controlled study. J Clin Psychiatry 1999;60:130-135;quiz 135-7.
79. Resch M, Szendei G, Haasz P. Bulimia from a gynecological view: hormonal changes. J Obstet Gynaecol. 2004;24:907–10.
80. Pike KM, Dogs M, Fichter MM, Tuschl RJ. Gonadotrophins, oestradiol and progesterone during the menstrual cycle in bulimia nervosa. Clin Endocrinol (Oxf.). 1988;29:265–70.
81. Schweiger U, Pike KM, Laessle RG, Fichter MM. Gonadotropin secretion in bulimia nervosa. J Clin Endocrinol Metab. 1992;74:1122–7.
82. Misra M, Miller KK, Cord J, Prabhakaran R, Herzog DB, Goldstein M, et al. Relationships between serum adipokines, insulin levels, and bone density in girls with anorexia nervosa. J Clin Endocrinol Metab. 2007;92:2046–52.
83. Kumai M, Tamai H, Fujii S, Nakagawa T, Aoki TT. Glucagon secretion in anorexia nervosa. Am J Clin Nutr. 1988;47:239–42.
84. Housova J, Anderlova K, Krizova J, Haluzikova D, Kremen J, Kumstyrova T, et al. Serum adiponectin and resistin concentrations in patients with restrictive and binge/purge form of anorexia nervosa and bulimia nervosa. J Clin Endocrinol Metab. 2005;90:1366–70.
85. Modan-Moses D, Stein D, Pariente C, Yaroslavsky A, Ram A, Faigin M, et al. Modulation of adiponectin and leptin during refeeding of female anorexia nervosa patients. J Clin Endocrinol Metab. 2007;92:1843–7.
86. Schwartz MW, Seeley RJ, Woods SC, Weigle DS, Campfield LA, Burn P, Baskin DG. Leptin increases hypothalamic pro-opiomelanocortin mRNA expression in the rostral arcuate nucleus. Diabetes. 1997;46:2119–23.
87. Germain N, Galusca B, Le Roux CW, Bossu C, Ghatei MA, Lang F, et al. Constitutional thinness and lean anorexia nervosa display opposite concentrations of peptide YY, glucagon-like peptide 1, ghrelin, and leptin. Am J Clin Nutr. 2007;85:967–71.
88. Munoz MT, Argente J. Anorexia nervosa in female adolescents: endocrine and bone mineral density disturbances. Eur J Endocrinol. 2002;147:275–86.
89. Cirmanova V, Bayer M, Starka L, Zajickova K. The effect of leptin on bone: an evolving concept of action. Physiol Res. 2008;57(Suppl 1):S143–51.
90. Misra M, Miller KK, Cord J, Prabhakaran R, Herzog DB, Goldstein M, et al. Relationships between serum adipokines, insulin levels, and bone density in girls with anorexia nervosa. J Clin Endocrinol Metab. 2007;92:2046–52.
91. Hebebrand J, Blum WF, Barth N, Coners H, Englaro P, Juul A, et al. Leptin levels in patients with anorexia nervosa are reduced in the acute stage and elevated upon short-term weight restoration. Mol Psychiatry. 1997;2:330–4.
92. Gendall KA, Kaye WH, Altemus M, McConaha CW, La Via MC. Leptin, neuropeptide Y, and peptide YY in long-term recovered eating disorder patients. Biol Psychiatry. 1999;46:292–9.
93. Misra M, Miller KK, Tsai P, Gallagher K, Lin A, Lee N, et al. Elevated peptide YY levels in adolescent girls with anorexia nervosa. J Clin Endocrinol Metab. 2006;91:1027–33.
94. Pfluger PT, Kampe J, Castaneda TR, Vahl T, D'Alessio DA, Kruthaupt T, et al. Effect of human body weight changes on circulating levels of peptide YY and peptide YY3-36. J Clin Endocrinol Metab. 2007;92:583–8.
95. Utz AL, Lawson EA, Misra M, Mickley D, Gleysteen S, Herzog DB, et al. Peptide YY (PYY) levels and bone mineral density (BMD) in women with anorexia nervosa. Bone. 2008;43:135–9.

96. Tolle V, Kadem M, Bluet-Pajot MT, Frere D, Foulon C, Bossu C, et al. Balance in ghrelin and leptin plasma levels in anorexia nervosa patients and constitutionally thin women. J Clin Endocrinol Metab. 2003;88:109–16.
97. Krassas GE. Endocrine abnormalities in anorexia nervosa. Pediatr Endocrinol Rev. 2003; 1:46–54.
98. Miljic D, Pekic S, Djurovic M, Doknic M, Milic N, Casanueva FF, et al. Ghrelin has partial or no effect on appetite, growth hormone, prolactin, and cortisol release in patients with anorexia nervosa. J Clin Endocrinol Metab. 2006;91:1491–5.
99. Otto B, Cuntz U, Fruehauf E, Wawarta R, Folwaczny C, Riepl RL, et al. Weight gain decreases elevated plasma ghrelin concentrations of patients with anorexia nervosa. Eur J Endocrinol. 2006;145:669–73.
100. Fairburn CG, Harrison PJ. Eating disorders. Lancet. 2003;361:407–16.
101. Steinhausen HC. The outcome of anorexia nervosa in the 20th century. Am J Psychiatry. 2002;159:1284–93.

Chapter 4
Skeletal Involvement in Eating Disorders

Nehama Zuckerman-Levin, Yael Latzer, Patricia E. Dunne and Ze'ev Hochberg

Abstract The effect of an eating disorder (ED) on bone health and the integrity of the skeletal structure, is an area of significant concern in terms of potential long-lasting, adverse consequences. Adolescence, in particular, represents a crucial developmental stage during which bone density accrues and peak bone mass is achieved. For this reason, EDs elevate the risk for bone loss among adolescents and young adults, and may jeopardize their ability to attain appropriate peak bone mass. Though some patients with EDs may not present with conspicuous symptomatology related to bone health, it is not uncommon for adolescents to develop stress fractures, kyphoscoliosis, or evidence height loss and for adults with EDs to suffer from bone pains and an increased incidence of fractures. In this chapter, we give an overview of the impact of eating disorder symptomatology on the skeletal system for both adults and adolescents with AN. A key characteristic of patients with AN is bone loss, which is evidenced by low bone turnover, greater osteoclastic (bone resorptive) activity as compared to osteoblasic (bone formation) activity, and deterioration in both trabecular and cortical bone, though particularly in the former. Factors that influence bone loss in AN include malnutrition and low weight, reduced fat mass, glucocorticoid excess, impairment of the GH-IGF1 axis, and insufficient levels of estrogen and androgen. On the other hand, in cases of bulimia nervosa (BN), bone loss occurs far less often and usually in patients with a history

N. Zuckerman-Levin (✉) · Y. Latzer
Eating Disorders Institute, Psychiatric Division,
Rambam Medical Center, Haifa, Israel
e-mail: zuckerln@netvision.net.il

Y. Latzer
Faculty of Social Welfare and Health Sciences,
University of Haifa, Haifa, Israel

P.E. Dunne
Department of Clinical & Counseling Psychology, Teachers College,
Columbia University, New York, NY, USA

Z. Hochberg
Rappaport Faculty of Medicine and Research Institute,
Technion-Israel Institute of Technology, Haifa, Israel

Y. Latzer and D. Stein (eds.), *Bio-Psycho-Social Contributions to Understanding Eating Disorders*, DOI 10.1007/978-3-319-32742-6_4

of low body weight or amenorrhea. From a treatment perspective, the most effective treatment for improving bone mineral density (BMD) is an increase in caloric intake, resulting in weight gain and resumption of menses. Other treatment modalities, such as those involving hormonal therapies, have not been found to have significant efficacy. Still, even in weight-restored patients with AN, long-lasting effects and permanent bone loss may result.

Introduction

Adolescence represents a unique and critical stage of development during which the accrual of bone density occurs and peak bone mass is attained. Individuals with eating disorders (EDs), however, face heightened risk for bone loss and, especially in cases of underweight, may fail to reach appropriate peak bone mass. Although a portion of patients with EDs may not exhibit characteristic symptoms, many more do, with adults reporting bone pain and an increased incidence of fractures and adolescents evidencing stress fractures, kyphoscoliosis and height loss [1]. In this chapter, we review current medical perspectives on the etiology of bone loss in patients with eating disorders, treatment approaches to preventing bone loss, and the effects of specific hormonal agents on the human skeletal system.

Characteristics of Bone Loss in Patients with ED

The significant bone loss observed in patients with Anorexia Nervosa (AN) is related to low bone turnover. Low bone turnover arises when osteoclastic (bone resorptive) activity and osteoblasic (bone formation) activity become imbalanced, such that the former far exceeds the later [2]. Thus, among these patients, bone resorption outpaces bone formation, resulting in bone loss. Notably, the mechanism involved in bone loss associated with AN differs from that of senile or glucocorticoid-related bone loss, which are effects of high bone turnover.

It is of great concern that bone loss in AN does not develop gradually over time, but rather, may ensue early on within the first 12 months of the eating disorder [3]. Once bone loss begins, it may progress with an average annual loss of 1 %, during a developmental stage in which normal bone minerals should be increasing [4].

Among patients with AN, trabecular bone is most susceptible to bone loss, however, it also effects cortical bone [5, 6] Results from volumetric measures performed on AN patients reveal decreases in the mineral content of the bone, as well as in size, which is measured according to vertebral body and femoral neck width [7].

Assessing Bone Health

The most common method of measuring Bone Mineral Density (BMD) is with Dual-Energy X-ray Absorptiometry (DEXA), which evaluates areal BMD. However, a significant limitation of this method is that it underestimates the measurement of BMD in short children and pre-pubertal adolescents. Consequently, DEXA underestimates the amount of bone loss in patients with AN. For this reason, other methods that permit bone structure to be assessed may be more appropriate options for evaluating bone health in patients with AN. Examples of such methods include Quantiative Computed Tomography (qCT), which measures 3-D volumetric BMD; quantitative US; and the newest form of technology, flat-panel volume CT. In terms of timing, it is recommended that evaluation of BMD in AN cases occur after 6–12 months of amenorrhea [8]. At the same time, bone metabolism can be gauged through an assessment of bone formation and bone resorption markers.

Clinical Presentation of Bone Loss in EDs

Research indicates that roughly half of adolescents with AN have age-corrected Z-scores of less than −1 at one or more skeletal sites, while 11 % obtain Z-scores below −2 [9]. Meanwhile, another study of adolescent girls with AN found that while total body DEXA was typically normal [10], over half of the girls had osteopenia and a quarter (25 %) evidenced osteoporosis at lumbar and femoral sites. These study results attest to the greater vulnerability of trabecular bones to bone loss, whereas cortical bones tend to be affected only in very severe cases [10]. On the other hand, in adolescent boys with AN, the hip and femoral neck bones are implicated more extensively as sites of cortical bone, than is the spine [11].

The consequences of AN as regards bone health are exacerbated by the fact that adolescence represents a developmental period in which bone accrual changes considerably and high bone turnover is commonly observed. Thus, AN in adolescence is characterized by impaired bone formation, which results from a decrease in the surrogate markers of bone formation, namely, serum osteocalcin and bone-specific alkaline phosphatase, relative to levels seen in healthy controls [2]. However, bone resorption markers in patients with AN have been found to be comparable to those in controls. Despite exhibiting normal BMD, assessments of flat-panel volume CT in adolescent girls with AN reveal abnormal trabecular structure when compared to normal-weight controls [12]. Patients who develop AN during adolescence are at particular risk for long-lasting and permanent deficits, given that the disease's onset frequently coincides with peak bone mass accrual. Even after a year of recovery, adolescent girls with AN may show persisting poor bone mineral accrual, as compared to the rapid bone accrual occurring in healthy controls [13].

Adults with AN also experience bone loss, as evidenced by elevated markers of resorption including N-teleopeptide and deoxypyrydoline, as well as decreased or normal bone formation markers such as osteocalcin [14]. Reduced BMD resulting in osteopenia is reported in up to 92 % of young adults with AN, while osteoporosis, in at least one site, occurs in 38–50 % [15]. Among men with AN, bone disease is less prevalent, but more severe, with 36 % experiencing osteopenia and 26 % osteoporosis [16, 17].

Compared to women with adult-onset AN, those who developed AN in adolescence have lower bone mass [6], independent of other variables that correlate with bone density (such as duration of amenorrhea or urinary cortisol excretion).

In cases of normal-weight Bulimia Nervosa (BN), low BMD is usually only seen among those patients with a history of low weight, menstrual disturbances, or amenorrhea [16, 18, 19]. The precise percentage of bone loss that occurs in BN is unknown, due to the heterogeneity of this group of patients.

The Pathogenesis of Bone Loss in ED

Numerous variables influence low BMD in patients with AN, including reduced caloric intake, low body weight, malnutrition, hypogonadism, thyroid function impairment, and low levels of PYY, Leptin and IGF1, in conjunction with elevated levels of circulating cortisol. Therefore, it is essential that treatment address all of these mechanisms, as correcting only one or several components is unlikely to stem bone loss.

A comprehensive examination of the aforementioned variables indicates that they largely fall into two categories, namely nutrition, and the hormonal milieu of EDs, which encompasses the endocrinological factors implicated in EDs. Significantly, these two categories are intertwined and exert influence over one another.

Nutrition

In both males and females with AN, nutritional markers such as low Body Mass Index (BMI), fat and lean body mass, and IGF1, are key determinants of low bone density [2, 9, 11, 13, 20]. The significance of these factors is consistent with the well-known health advantages of weight loading and muscle pull on bone. Accordingly, nutritional rehabilitation, which has an anabolic effect on bone metabolism, is the basis of treatment for osteopenia and osteoporosis in AN. Meanwhile, weight gain is linked to the recovery of bone formation [13, 21], because it promotes normalization of bone turnover markers and increases IGF1 levels. Significantly, menses must be resumed before bone resorption markers can be decelerated to a point at which they resemble those in healthy controls [21].

Although Calcium and Vitamin D are both vital to bone mineralization, patients with AN frequently have adequate levels of these nutrients, hence supplementation with these nutrients in such patients is not associated with improved bone density [13].

Hormonal Milieu of Eating Disorders

Estrogens—Estrogens, which are bone resorptive, inhibit the osteoclast—mediated destruction of bone by binding to the RANK-RANKL system. Estrogens stimulate osteoclast and inhibit osteocyte apoptosis, while maintaining osteocyte viability [22]. Given that estrogen-deficient states are characterized by elevated markers of bone resorption, it follows then that the longer the duration of amenorrhea, the greater the BMD decrease in women with AN [6, 23]. By comparison, women with AN evidence more severe bone loss than healthy women who have functional hypothalamic amenorrhea [23]. Just as weight gain in adults with AN is accompanied by improved hip BMD, the resumption of menses impacts spine BMD, thereby illustrating the influence of estrogen on trabecular bone density [24].

Yet in spite of estrogen's advantageous effects on bone preservation, estrogen therapy on its own will not effectively increase bone density in adolescents or adults with AN [25–27] until weight has been restored [21]. Indeed, a subgroup of low-weight eumenorrheic women exhibited low bone density, even though they showed normal gonadal function and higher IGFI levels [28]. Troublingly, it may be the case that high-dose estrogens at levels on par with those commonly found in oral contraceptives, may further diminish IGF1 levels.

Androgens—Bone health in AN is also influenced by androgen deficiency. Oral contraceptives are also known to decrease androgen levels, which is particularly problematic in patients with AN who already exhibit androgen deficiency. In turn, reduced levels of androgens predict lower BMD [29]. While there is some indication that short-term replacement therapy with testosterone or DHEAS can improve certain bone turnover markers in women with AN [30, 31], once weight gain in this particular study's DHEAS-treated women was taken into account, any significant improvement in BMD was no longer apparent [31].

Cortisol—Patients with AN have higher than normal levels of serum cortisol, which advances bone loss by stimulating osteoclast activity and inhibiting osteoblast activity. Conversely, in healthy individuals, estrogen shields osteoblasts from the effects of cortisol. Furthermore, cortisol influences calcium metabolism and the GH-IGFI axis. As a result, urinary free cortisol in patients with AN is inversely correlated with spine BMD [6], whereas serum cortisol is inversely correlated with markers of bone formation [32]. Most importantly, cortisol excess is linked to severity of bone loss in AN [33].

GH resistance and IGF1 deficiency—Both GH resistance and IGFI deficiency play a role in reducing BMD in AN, with GH acting via IGF1 and exerting an anabolic effect on bone, and low levels of IGF1 reducing osteocalcin levels and impacting osteoblast function [27]. Unlike healthy adolescent girls, in whom GH levels predict bone turnover markers, this is not the case in adolescent girls with AN [34]. In addition, among girls with AN, low levels of IGF1 predict lower BMD and bone formation markers [13]. That said, research involving adult women with AN who were administered a combined IGFI—estrogen treatment, showed an increase in spine BMD and bone formation markers, along with a decrease in bone resorption markers [27].

Hypothalamic-pituitary-thyroid axis—This axis is essential to skeletal development, the accumulation of peak bone mass, and the regulation of bone turnover in adults. It is suspected that low triiodothyronine may disrupt normal bone metabolism in patients with AN [35]. Yet although thyroid hormones have an anabolic effect on bone and generate local IGF1 secretion, thyroid replacement therapy has not been found to ameliorate AN-related osteopenia.

Osteoprotegerin (OPG)—OPG, which is a cytokine receptor and a member of the TNF receptor superfamily, maintains bone density by stimulating osteoclast apoptosis and inhibiting osteoclast differentiation and activation. It is stimulated in vivo by estrogens. AN is associated with elevated OPG levels, which in turn, negatively correlate with BMI, estradiol, IGF1, and Leptin [36]. It has been hypothesized that a compensatory mechanism for low weight and estrogens may exist in patients with AN, resulting in increased levels of OPG [36].

Leptin—Leptin has been found to exert both central and peripheral, and anabolic and adverse effects on bone [37]. Leptin also regulates the processes involved in bone remodeling, exhibiting a direct stimulatory effect on osteoblast differentiation and bone formation, and an indirect effect through the hypothalamus (ventromedial nucleus) in the sympathetic nervous system [38, 39]. Patients with AN are frequently deficient in Leptin, which contributes to low bone mass [40]. Further research is needed to determine what role, if any, Leptin may play in treating bone loss related to EDs.

Adiponectin—Adiponectin levels inversely predict bone density in adolescents with AN [40]. As such, elevated adiponectin levels like those seen in patients with AN, may contribute to reduced BMD by increasing osteoclast activity.

PYY Levels—which are high in individuals with AN, may promote bone loss on account of their association with low levels of bone turnover markers [41]. Along these lines, high PYY levels in adults with AN predicts lower bone density [42]. An inverse correlation such as that between PYY levels and bone turnover markers aligns with findings from rodent studies that demonstrate increased osteoblastic activity and selective deletion of the Y2 receptor [43].

Ghrelin—While Ghrelin is known to stimulate osteoblast proliferation and differentiation [44], the few available in vivo studies of the hormone indicate that it is only weakly connected to BMD. The effects of reduced Ghrelin—Obestatin (another gastric hormone) ratio on bone health in patients with AN are currently under investigation.

Consequences of Bone Loss Due to an ED

Alongside bone mineral accrual, growth represents another principal concern with regards to bone loss in adolescence. Factors that determine whether adolescents with AN will successfully attain predicted height include the age and pubertal stage of the patient at the time of the disease's onset, the degree of bone age delay, and both the duration and severity of AN in a given case [1, 45]. In instances in which an adolescent fails to attain peak bone mass, consequences may include stress fractures in adolescence or young adulthood [46] or osteoporotic fractures later in life. Elevated fracture rates have been reported in cases of AN, BN, and Eating Disorders Not Otherwise Specified (EDNOS) [47]. Specifically, patients with AN who have experienced amenorrhea in excess of 6 years, are seven times more likely to suffer a fracture [47], while studies of long-term outcome in patients with AN demonstrate that 44 % of patients who are unrecovered at 11.7 years follow-up, are osteoporotic [48]. Moreover, results from one longitudinal study showed that 40 years after receiving a diagnosis of AN, the cumulative incidence of any fracture was 57 % [49].

Treatments for Bone Loss in EDs

Physical activity, specifically weight-bearing exercise, is known to have a significant influence on bone health and contributes to an increase in peak BMD [50]. Yet in cases of AN, in which individuals frequently evidence malnourishment, the recommendation of physical activity as a prescriptive measure is both controversial and arguably, unethical. Accordingly, the particular history of a patient with AN, including past experiences with over-exercising, must be taken into account when weighing such a recommendation [51]. In addition, these concerns should be discussed thoroughly with the patient.

Biophosphonates, which reduce bone turnover by decreasing bone resorption through osteoclasts, have been studied only sparingly. That said, results from one study in which patients with AN were treated with risedronate, showed that bone density had increased [52]. However, this group of drugs has a strong affinity to bone, as is evidenced by their absorption into its matrix, therefore they are not recommended as a treatment for low-turnover bone loss among cases of AN.

Cannabinoids play a key role in the regulation of eating behavior within the central nervous system, as well as in adipose and intestine tissue. In connection with regulating food consumption, Cannabinoids interact with Ghrelin, Leptin, and also Melancortins. However, based on results from the mere handful of studies conducted that have investigated the use of cannabinoids in patients with AN, they have not been found to stimulate appetite or induce weight gain in any significant capacity [53].

Long-Term Outcome and Implications

Bone loss represents one of the most harmful and irreversible consequences of EDs. The fact that individuals who successfully regain weight, resume menses, and reestablish nutritional health, may still evidence persisting bone loss or suffer long-term effects, is especially disturbing [13, 18, 54]. Overall outcome may be better among patients who begin weight-gain focused nutrition treatment and psychotherapy early on in the course of their disease and who continue treatment. Conversely, prognostic indicators such as prolonged course and chronicity, extremely low body weight, and early onset of ED in adolescence prior to the attainment of peak bone mass, are associated with poorer outcome and longer-term impairment. Notably, nutritional rehabilitation is not just essential to recovery in its own right, as it also helps ensure that other psychotherapies have their maximum positive effect.

Take home points

- Adolescence represents a critical period of development during which bone density increases and peak bone mass is attained.
- Adolescents and young adults who develop an ED are at heightened risk for bone loss or failure to attain age-appropriate peak bone mass, which in turn, increases their susceptibility to stress fractures, kyphoscoliosis and height loss.
- Adults with EDs may experience bone pain and on the whole, report an increased incidence of fractures.
- Individuals with AN demonstrate low bone turnover, characterized by less osteoblasic (bone formation) activity occuring relative to osteoclastic (bone resorptive) activity, and bone loss ensues in the trabecular bone, principally, but may also occur in the cortical bone.
- Malnourishment, which is most evident in patients with AN, can result in osteopenia or osteoporosis, depending on its degree of severity and length of duration.
- Individuals with BN, who are normal weight, typically do not show low BMD unless they have a past history of low weight or amenorrhea.
- Numerous factors have been determined to play a role in bone loss associated with AN, some of which include malnutrition and low weight, reduced fat mass, estrogen and androgen deficiency, impaired GH-IGF1 axis, and glucocorticoid excess.
- The most effective means of improving BMD is through increased caloric intake, weight gain and the resumption of menses, whereas other treatment modalities involving hormonal therapies have demonstrated only limited efficacy.
- Even after recovery and weight gain following AN, bone loss caused by the disease may not be completely reversible and the damage may have lasting effects.

References

1. Modan-Moses D, Yaroslavsky A, Novikov I, Segev S, Toledano A, Miterany E, Stein D. Stunting of growth as a major feature of anorexia nervosa in male adolescents. Pediatrics. 2003;111:270–6.
2. Soyka LA, Grinspoon S, Levitsky LL, Herzog DB, Kilbanski A. The effects of anorexia nervosa on bone metabolism in female adolescents. J Clin Endocrinol Metab. 1999;84:4489–96.
3. Wong JC, Lewindon P, Mortimer R, Shepherd R. Bone mineral density in adolescent females with recently diagnosed anorexia nervosa. Int J Eat Disord. 2001;29:11–6.
4. Serafinowicz E, Wasikowa R, Iwanicka Z, Jedrzejuk D. Bone metabolism in adolescent girls with short course of anorexia nervosa. Endokrynol Diabetol Chor Przemiany Materii Wieku Rozw. 2003;9:67–71.
5. Milos G, Spindler A, Ruegsegger P, Seifert B, Muhlebach S, Uebelhart D, Hauselmann HJ. Cortical and trabecular bone density and structure in anorexia nervosa. Osteoporos Int. 2005;16:783–90.
6. Biller BM, Saxe V, Herzog DB, Rosenthal DI, Holzman S, Klibanski A. Mechanisms of osteoporosis in adult and adolescent women with anorexia nervosa. J Clin Endocrinol Metab. 1989;68:548–54.
7. Karlsson MK, Weigall SJ, Duan Y, Seeman E. Bone size and volumetric density in women with anorexia nervosa receiving estrogen replacement therapy and in women recovered from anorexia nervosa. J Clin Endocrinol Metab. 2000;85:3177–82.
8. Castro J, Lazaro L, Pons F, Halperin I, Toro J. Predictors of bone mineral density reduction in adolescents with anorexia nervosa. J Am Acad Child Adolesc Psychiatry. 2000;39:1365–70.
9. Misra M, Aggarwal A, Miller KK, Almazan C, Worley M, Soyka LA, et al. Effects of anorexia nervosa on clinical, hematologic, biochemical, and bone density parameters in community-dwelling adolescent girls. Pediatrics. 2004;114:1574–83.
10. Pafumi C, Ciotta L, Farina M, Bosco P, Chiarenza M, Pernicone G, et al. Evaluation of bone mass in young amenorrheic women with anorexia nervosa. Minerva Ginecol. 2002;54:487–91.
11. Misra M, Katzman DK, Clarke H, Snelgrove D, Brigham K, Miller KK, Klibanski A. Hip structural analysis in adolescent boys with anorexia nervosa and controls. J Clin Endocrinol Metab. 2013;98(7):2952–8. doi:10.1210/jc.2013-1457 Epub 2013 May 7.
12. Bredella MA, Misra M, Miller KK, Madisch I, Sarwar A, Cheung A, et al. Distal radius in adolescent girls with anorexia nervosa: trabecular structure analysis with high-resolution flat-panel volume CT. Radiology. 2008;249:938–46.
13. Soyka LA, Misra M, Frenchman A, Miller KK, Grinspoon S, Schoenfeld DA, Kilbanski A. Abnormal bone mineral accrual in adolescent girls with anorexia nervosa. J Clin Endocrinol Metab. 2002;87:4177–85.
14. Lennkh C, de Zwaan M, Bailer U, Strnad A, Nagy C, El-Giamal N, et al. Osteopenia in anorexia nervosa: specific mechanisms of bone loss. J Psychiatr Res. 1999;33:349–56.
15. Grinspoon S, Thomas E, Pitts S, Gross E, Mickley D, Miller K, et al. Prevalence and predictive factors for regional osteopenia in women with anorexia nervosa. Ann Intern Med. 2000;133:790–4.
16. Mehler PS, Sabel AL, Watson T, Andersen AE. High risk of osteoporosis in male patients with eating disorders. Int J Eat Disord. 2008;41:666–72.
17. Andersen AE, Watson T, Schlechte J. Osteoporosis and osteopenia in men with eating disorders. Lancet. 2000;355:1967–8.
18. Zipfel S, Seibel MJ, Lowe B, Beumont PJ, Kasperk C, Herzog W. Osteoporosis in eating disorders: a follow-up study of patients with anorexia and bulimia nervosa. J Clin Endocrinol Metab. 2001;86:5227–33.
19. Naessen S, Carlstrom K, Glant R, Jacobsson H, Hirschberg AL. Bone mineral density in bulimic women–influence of endocrine factors and previous anorexia. Eur J Endocrinol. 2006;155:245–51.

20. Hotta M, Fukuda I, Sato K, Hizuka N, Shibasaki T, Takano K. The relationship between bone turnover and body weight, serum insulin-like growth factor (IGF) I, and serum IGF-binding protein levels in patients with anorexia nervosa. J Clin Endocrinol Metab. 2000;85:200–6.
21. Dominguez J, Goodman L, Gupta SS, Mayer L, Etu SF, Walsh BT, et al. Treatment of anorexia nervosa is associated with increases in bone mineral density, and recovery is a biphasic process involving both nutrition and return of menses. Am J Clin Nutr. 2007;86:92–9.
22. Riggs BL. The mechanisms of estrogen regulation of bone resorption. J Clin Invest. 2000;106:1203–4.
23. Grinspoon S, Miller K, Coyle C, Krempin J, Armstrong C, Pitts S, et al. Severity of osteopenia in estrogen-deficient women with anorexia nervosa and hypothalamic amenorrhea. J Clin Endocrinol Metab. 1999;84:2049–55.
24. Miller KK, Lee EE, Lawson EA, Misra M, Minihan J, Grinspoon SK, et al. Determinants of skeletal loss and recovery in anorexia nervosa. J Clin Endocrinol Metab. 2006;91:2931–7.
25. Klibanski A, Biller BM, Schoenfeld DA, Herzog DB, Saxe VC. The effects of estrogen administration on trabecular bone loss in young women with anorexia nervosa. J Clin Endocrinol Metab. 1995;80:898–904.
26. Golden NH, Lanzkowsky L, Schebendach J, Palestro CJ, Jacobson M, Shenker IR. The effect of estrogen-progestin treatment on bone mineral density in anorexia nervosa. J Pediatr Adolesc Gynecol. 2002;15:135–43.
27. Grinspoon S, Thomas L, Miller K, Herzog D, Klibanski A. Effects of recombinant human IGF-I and oral contraceptive administration on bone density in anorexia nervosa. J Clin Endocrinol Metab. 2002;87:2883–91.
28. Miller KK, Grinspoon S, Gleysteen S, Grieco KA, Ciampa J, Breu J, et al. Preservation of neuroendocrine control of reproductive function despite severe undernutrition. J Clin Endocrinol Metab. 2004;89:4434–8.
29. Miller KK, Lawson EA, Mathur V, Wexler TL, Meenaghan E, Misra M, et al. Androgens in women with anorexia nervosa and normal-weight women with hypothalamic amenorrhea. J Clin Endocrinol Metab. 2007;92:1334–9.
30. Miller KK, Grieco KA, Klibanski A. Testosterone administration in women with anorexia nervosa. J Clin Endocrinol Metab. 2005;90:1428–33.
31. Gordon CM, Grace E, Emans SJ, Feldman HA, Goodman E, Becker KA, et al. Effects of oral dehydroepiandrosterone on bone density in young women with anorexia nervosa: a randomized trial. J Clin Endocrinol Metab. 2002;87:4935–41.
32. Misra M, Miller KK, Almazan C, Ramaswamy K, Lapcharoensap W, Worley M, et al. Alterations in cortisol secretory dynamics in adolescent girls with anorexia nervosa and effects on bone metabolism. J Clin Endocrinol Metab. 2004;89:4972–80.
33. Lawson EA, Donoho D, Miller KK, Misra M, Meenaghan E, Lydecker J, et al. Hypercortisolemia is associated with severity of bone loss and depression in hypothalamic amenorrhea and anorexia nervosa. J Clin Endocrinol Metab. 2009;94:4710–6.
34. Misra M, Miller KK, Bjornson J, Hackman A, Aggarwal A, Chung J, et al. Alterations in growth hormone secretory dynamics in adolescent girls with anorexia nervosa and effects on bone metabolism. J Clin Endocrinol Metab. 2003;88:5615–23.
35. Galusca B, Bossu C, Germain N, Kadem M, Frere D, Lafage-Proust MH, et al. Age-related differences in hormonal and nutritional impact on lean anorexia nervosa bone turnover uncoupling. Osteoporos Int. 2006;17:888–96.
36. Ohwada R, Hotta M, Sato K, Shibasaki T, Takano K. The relationship between serum levels of estradiol and osteoprotegerin in patients with anorexia nervosa. Endocr J. 2007;54:953–9.
37. Cirmanova V, Bayer M, Starka L, Zajickova K. The effect of leptin on bone: an evolving concept of action. Physiol Res. 2008;57(Suppl 1):S143–51.
38. Isaia GC, D'Amelio P, Di Bella S, Tamone C. Is leptin the link between fat and bone mass? J Endocrinol Invest. 2005;28(Suppl 10):61–5.
39. Cohen MM. Role of leptin in regulating appetite, neuroendocrine function, and bone remodeling. Am J Med Genet A. 2006;140:515–24.

40. Misra M, Miller KK, Cord J, Prabhakaran R, Herzog DB, Goldstein M, et al. Relationships between serum adipokines, insulin levels, and bone density in girls with anorexia nervosa. J Clin Endocrinol Metab. 2007;92:2046–52.
41. Misra M, Miller KK, Cord J, Prabhakaran R, Herzog DB, Goldstein M, et al. Elevated peptide YY levels in adolescent girls with anorexia nervosa. J Clin Endocrinol Metab. 2006;91:1027–33.
42. Utz AL, Lawson EA, Misra M, Mickley D, Gleysteen S, Herzog DB, et al. Peptide YY (PYY) levels and bone mineral density (BMD) in women with anorexia nervosa. Bone. 2008;43:135–9.
43. Baldock PA, Sainsbury A, Couzens M, Enriquez RF, Thomas GP, Gardiner EM, Herzog H. Hypothalamic Y2 receptors regulate bone formation. J Clin Invest. 2002;109:915–21.
44. Fukushima N, Hanada R, Teranishi H, Fukue Y, Tachibana T, Ishikawa H, et al. Ghrelin directly regulates bone formation. J Bone Miner Res. 2005;20:790–8.
45. Prabhakaran R, Misra M, Miller KK, Kruczek K, Sundaralingam S, Herzog DB, et al. Determinants of height in adolescent girls with anorexia nervosa. Pediatrics. 2008;121:e1517–23.
46. Baum ML, Kramer EL, Sanger JJ, Pena A. Stress fractures and reduced bone mineral density with prior anorexia nervosa. J Nucl Med. 1987;28:1506–7.
47. Vestergaard P, Emborg C, Stoving RK, Hagen C, Mosekilde L, Brixen K. Fractures in patients with anorexia nervosa, bulimia nervosa, and other eating disorders–a nationwide register study. Int J Eat Disord. 2002;32:301–8.
48. Herzog W, Minne H, Deter C, Leidig G, Schellberg D, Wuster C, et al. Outcome of bone mineral density in anorexia nervosa patients 11.7 years after first admission. J Bone Miner Res. 1993;8:597–605.
49. Lucas AR, Melton LJ, Crowson CS, O'Fallon WM. Long-term fracture risk among women with anorexia nervosa: a population-based cohort study. Mayo Clin Proc. 1999;74:972–7.
50. Lloyd T, Chinchilli VM, Johnson-Rollings N, Kieselhorst K, Eggli DF, Marcus R. Adult female hip bone density reflects teenage sports-exercise patterns but not teenage calcium intake. Pediatrics. 2000;106:40–4.
51. Putukian M. The female athlete triad. Clin Sports Med. 1998;17:675–96.
52. Miller KK, Grieco KA, Mulder J, Grinspoon S, Mickley D, Yehezkel R, et al. Effects of risedronate on bone density in anorexia nervosa. J Clin Endocrinol Metab. 2004;89:3903–6.
53. Stoving RK, Andries A, Brixen K, Flyvbjerg A, Horder K, Frystyk J. Leptin, ghrelin, and endocannabinoids: potential therapeutic targets in anorexia nervosa. J Psychiatr Res. 2009;43:671–9.
54. Rigotti NA, Nussbaum SR, Herzog DB, Neer RM. Osteoporosis in women with anorexia nervosa. N Engl J Med. 1984;311:1601–6.

Part II
Psychological Issues

Chapter 5
Suicidal Behavior in Eating Disorders

Lisa Rachelle Riso Lilenfeld

Abstract Anorexia nervosa has the highest mortality rate of any psychiatric illness, with suicide being the second leading cause of death. In addition to frank suicide attempts (some of which are premeditated and some of which are impulsive), many individuals with eating disorders engage in other intentional forms of self-injury, especially those individuals with purging symptomatology. In fact, those who use multiple purging strategies are especially likely to attempt suicide. Prospective predictors of suicidality in this population include having a co-morbid substance use disorder and engaging in laxative abuse. In addition, multiple forms of impulsive behavior are common among those individuals with eating disorders who have attempted suicide. Clinicians working with an eating disordered population must be aware of the high risk of suicidality in order to appropriately assess for, and monitor this risk vigilantly throughout treatment, because we now know that heightened suicide risk may continue even after eating disorder symptoms begin to improve. Thus, careful assessment of suicidal ideation, as well as degree of lethality and intent to die, must be part of the initial, as well as ongoing assessment, in the treatment of individuals with eating disorders.

Scope of the Problem

Mortality

Individuals suffering from eating disorders are often the least desirable patients with whom clinicians wish to work. Undoubtedly, one reason is their resistance to change, particularly among those with anorexia nervosa [1]. Another reason is the high lethality of the condition, especially among those with anorexia nervosa.

L.R.R. Lilenfeld (✉)
Clinical Psychology Program, American School of Professional Psychology
at Argosy University, Washington D.C., 1550 Wilson Boulevard, Suite 600,
Arlington, VA 22209, USA
e-mail: LLilenfeld@argosy.edu

Y. Latzer and D. Stein (eds.), *Bio-Psycho-Social Contributions to Understanding Eating Disorders*, DOI 10.1007/978-3-319-32742-6_5

Indeed, anorexia nervosa appears to have the highest death rate of any psychiatric illness [2]. One reason for mortality is complications of the eating disorder itself, such as organ failure. However, another frequent cause of mortality is suicide, which is thought to be the second leading cause of death among those with anorexia nervosa [2]. It had been previously believed that when people die from the illness, it was almost always due to the effects of starvation itself. This assumption has now been challenged, based upon recent studies documenting extremely elevated rates of suicide in this population [e.g., 3, 4].

Standardized mortality ratio refers to the number of observed deaths divided by the number of expected deaths [5], providing an estimate of the risk of death in a particular group of people. While suicide attempts are frequent among individuals with bulimia nervosa [6], the standardized mortality ratios for bulimia nervosa and binge eating disorder appear nonsignificant [7]. By contrast, nearly all studies of anorexia nervosa have found significantly increased standardized mortality ratios [8–23] with one exception where nonreferred patients were studied and no excess mortality was found [24]. All of the other standardized mortality ratios have ranged from 2.9 to 17.8. A recent large epidemiological cohort study of individuals with various eating disorders, followed for 7–10 years, found a standardized mortality ratio of 10.5 for anorexia nervosa specifically [25]. Sullivan [2] similarly concluded from his meta-analysis that the aggregate annual mortality rate associated with anorexia nervosa is more than 12 times higher than the annual death rate due to all causes of death for females 15–24 years of age in the general population. Specifically, he found that the mortality rate for anorexia nervosa was 5.6 % per decade. In addition, Sullivan [2] found that the aggregate annual mortality rate associated with anorexia nervosa is more than twice what was found among a national study group of female psychiatric inpatients between the ages of 10 and 39. More recently, Steinhausen [26] has estimated an almost 18-fold increase in mortality among those with anorexia nervosa. Finally and sadly, a 57-fold greater risk of death from suicide for individuals with anorexia nervosa, relative to an age-matched cohort from the general population, has been found [11].

It should be noted that as with alcohol use disorders, eating disorders continue to have a similar social stigma and, therefore, it is quite likely that reference to an eating disorder may not be mentioned on a death certificate, particularly in the context of a documented suicide [27]. This tendency to underreport eating disorders on death certificates may, in fact, have contributed to the mistaken assumption by many that these conditions are relatively infrequent and rarely fatal.

Rates and Nature of Suicidality

In a meta-analysis of suicide in anorexia nervosa, Pompili et al. [4] examined nine studies which included 1,538 patients, with a range of follow-up from 5 to 23 years. In all studies [9, 15, 19–21, 28], the Aberdeen cohort of Crisp et al. [22] but one (the St. George's cohort of Crisp et al. [22]), the expected suicides in a year among individuals with anorexia nervosa was significantly greater than the expected suicides in a year among the general population, aged 14–25 years. In fact, averaging across these studies, the expected number of suicides was 8 times greater among a population of individuals with anorexia nervosa compared to those aged 14–25 in the general population.

The nature of the suicide attempts is indeed serious in most of these cases. Bulik et al. [29] found that among 69 individuals with eating disorders had a history of at least one suicide attempt, 55 % required medical attention for their most serious attempt and 46 % were hospitalized. With regard to intent, notably 78 % expressed a wish to die and 57 % believed that they actually would die. Moderate (e.g., a brief period of unconsciousness) or extreme (e.g., prolonged coma) severity of the attempt was reported in 54 % of those who attempted suicide. Finally and of great important to clinicians working with this population, 49 % were reported to have been impulsive acts, while 25 % were somewhat premeditated, and another 25 % were completely premeditated. Thus, many of these suicide attempts represent explicit wishes to die with expectations of death and serious medical consequences; half are planful while half are impulsive.

Other Parasuicidal Behavior

In addition to suicide attempts, yet another reason for many clinicians' reticence to work with this population is the frequent occurrence of parasuicidal behavior, which encompasses both frank suicide attempts, as well as intentional self-injury, with or without an explicit intent to die [30]. This behavior is most commonly found among individuals with purging symptomatology [e.g., 31, 32] and indeed, some conceptualize the compensatory behavior found in the purging subtype of bulimia nervosa to be a form of deliberate self-harm. Others have proposed dividing such intentional self-injurious behavior into "impulsive" (e.g., skin cutting and burning) and "compulsive" (e.g., severe nail biting) categories [e.g., 33]. Compulsive parasuicidal behavior has been described as habitual and repetitive, while impulsive parasuicidal behavior has been described as episodic and providing some gratification beyond tension relief [33]. The presence of impulsive self-injurious behavior has been associated with a history of sexual abuse and laxative abuse. By contrast, compulsive self-injurious behavior has been associated with self-induced vomiting. Both types of self-injurious behavior have been associated with poor interoceptive awareness, that is, problems in accurately recognizing and attending to various internal states [33].

Finally, some have noted that patients with purging behavior are also more likely to actually commit suicide than those without purging behavior [e.g., 34]. Yet, most studies of individuals with bulimia nervosa have found fewer completed suicides than that which has been observed with anorexia nervosa [35]. However, the highest rates of other parasuicidal behavior, including impulsive self-injury, are indeed found among those with a diagnosis of bulimia nervosa [e.g., 36]; again, the strongest predictor of such behavior within this diagnostic category is the presence of purging behavior [e.g., 33].

Predictors of Suicidality

Prospective Predictors of Suicidality Among Adults

Franko et al. [37] conducted one of the few prospective studies of suicidality among individuals with eating disorders. They studied 246 women with anorexia nervosa and bulimia nervosa over an 8 year period of time. They found that women with anorexia nervosa were more likely to attempt suicide than women with bulimia nervosa. They also found that the severity of drug use over the course of the study predicted suicide among women with anorexia nervosa, specifically. Interestingly, one of the strongest and most consistent predictors of a fatal outcome among those with anorexia nervosa (due to suicide and other causes of death) was severity of alcohol use during the *follow-up* period [11]. Importantly for clinicians to note, one-third of these women with alcoholism who ultimately died had no history of any alcohol use disorder at the initial assessment. There are conflicting data regarding to what extent co-morbid major depressive disorder or severity of depression predict whether women with anorexia nervosa are likely to attempt suicide [37, 38].

With regard to predicting suicide attempts in bulimia nervosa, specific predictors have been found to include a history of drug use disorder and the use of laxatives [37]. In an attempt to isolate the psychopathology of bulimia nervosa apart from depression in predicting suicide attempts, Nickel et al. [39] conducted a prospective study of 28 women with purging-type bulimia nervosa and no co-morbid major depression, as well as 126 women with major depression and no eating disorder, all of whom were recruited from the community, inpatient, and outpatient settings and had attempted suicide during the subsequent 12 month period. It was found that the non-depressed bulimic women were more likely to have been beaten, sexually abused, separated from their parents for 6 weeks or longer during early childhood, abused various substances, and have higher levels of anger, compared to women with major depression and no eating disorder who also had attempted suicide. Thus, the risk factors for suicide attempts among those with bulimia nervosa in comparison with those who have major depression are different, and may indicate a different causal pathway to the endpoint of attempting to end one's life.

Prospective Predictors of Suicidality Among Adolescents

Another prospective study, this one of adolescents, found that extreme and unhealthy weight control behaviors (i.e., diet pill use, self-induced vomiting, use of laxatives or diuretics) predicted suicide attempts among young women (but not young men) 5 years later, even after taking into account depressive symptoms at that later time point [40]. These findings indicate that such early disordered eating behavior may be a risk marker for later suicidality.

Correlates of Suicidality

Eating Disorder Symptomatology

Suicide attempts are more likely to occur among those with purging symptomatology, in the context of either an anorexic or bulimic diagnosis [31, 32, 41, 42]. Those with multiple purging strategies may also be especially likely to have engaged in suicide attempts [31, 42].

Abuse History and Personality Traits

Other clinical correlates of suicidality among those with eating disorders are a history of physical or sexual abuse [32, 36, 43], as well as certain personality traits, including high levels of the temperamental traits of persistence (i.e., perfectionistic) and harm avoidance (i.e., fearful and pessimistic), low levels of the character trait of self-directedness (i.e., poor impulse control, associated with personality disorders), and high levels of the character trait of self-transcendence (i.e., spiritual and idealistic, may indicate a tendency toward dissociation or disconnectedness; [e.g., 38]).

In addition, impulsivity is a common theme among those individuals with eating disorders who have had at least one suicide attempt [e.g., 6]. The nature of the impulsivity may be primarily cognitive and center around the tendency to make quick decisions [29]. Multiple impulsive behaviors among those with an eating disorder and suicide histories have been noted, including impulsive substance use, recurrent shoplifting, sexual promiscuity, and physical aggression toward others [29, 42, 44, 45]. These patients are often referred to as "multi-impulsive" [44] and appear more likely to have a history of sexual abuse, poorer occupational and social functioning, and are more likely to have borderline and other cluster B personality disorders [44, 46, 47].

Co-morbid Psychopathology

Those individuals with eating disorders who have had one or more suicide attempts have also been found to have more significant histories of specific types of co-morbid psychopathology, namely substance use disorders and anxiety disorders, particularly panic disorder and post-traumatic stress disorder [29], as well as more significant mood disorder histories [e.g., 6]. Differences in the onset pattern of co-morbid disorders among eating disordered women with and without a history of parasuicide has been examined by one group of researchers, with the purpose of examining potential etiologic differences between the two groups [48]. It was found that the average age of onset of major depression and anxiety disorders occurred at a younger age in the group of 27 women with eating disorders who also had a history of suicide attempts and other forms of parasuicide, compared to the group of 27 women with comparable eating disorders but no suicidality history. In addition, the onset of major depression was more likely to occur before the eating disorder in the parasuicidal group in contrast to the nonparasuicidal group where depression almost never preceded the eating disorder. Thus, it is possible that the eating disorder is more likely to be secondary to a mood disturbance in women with histories of parasuicide. That is, depression may be a preexisting and potentially important etiological factor in the development of an eating disorder in this group. By contrast, major depression may be a consequence of a primary eating disorder among those with no history of parasuicide [48].

Treatment Implications

Ongoing Assessment

Clinicians working with this population should be made aware of the high risk of suicide and parasuicide among individuals with eating disorders. Therefore, a thorough suicide assessment should be conducted for those with current and past histories of eating disorders. Importantly, because suicide risk may be ongoing and occur even after eating disorder symptoms show some improvement, vigilant assessment must be an ongoing process.

History of Anorexia Nervosa

An interesting finding of great clinical importance is that there may be a very high risk of frank suicide, rather than risk for death by malnutrition, for those patients who have a *history* of anorexia nervosa [3]. Instead, these individuals were most often found to be suffering from another significant and chronic form of an eating disorder, yet at a somewhat more normal body weight. The study by Crisp et al. [3] found that among those with a past history of anorexia nervosa who died, 58 % died from suicide, while none died from malnutrition. By contrast, those with a current anorexia nervosa diagnosis were more likely to have died from malnutrition (41 % of all deaths) than suicide (24 % of all deaths). Therefore, a clinician must be aware of all of the risk factors for suicide in this population, and be particularly vigilant when a number of these factors are present in an individual with a chronic illness course and some other current form of eating disorder, but a history of anorexia nervosa.

Illness Duration

Clinicians in the field already know that the longer the duration of illness, the worse the outcome [26]. Additional relevant findings to bear in mind come from the Mayo clinic, where data over a 50 year period of time (1938–1984) were examined. A mortality rate of 5 % among individuals with anorexia nervosa when the duration of illness was 4 to 5 years was found, but a mortality rate of 15–20 % was found when the duration of illness was between 20 and 30 years [49].

Features Associated with Fatal Outcome

In addition to longer duration of illness, it is important for clinicians to keep in mind that some other features associated with a fatal outcome are bingeing and purging, co-morbid substance abuse and co-morbid mood disorders [e.g., 15]. Given the very serious nature of most of these suicidal episodes [29], careful assessment of not only suicidal ideation, but also level of lethality and intention to die, should be a standard part of the initial and ongoing assessment in the treatment of individuals with eating disorders. In addition, based upon the finding that severity of problematic alcohol use was one of the strongest and most consistent predictors of a fatal outcome for those with anorexia nervosa [11], alcohol use must be monitored closely throughout treatment.

Functions of Suicidal Behavior

Lilenfeld et al. [50] have preliminary unpublished data examining the function of suicide attempts and other parasuicidal acts among 27 individuals who currently, or previously, had received treatment for an eating disorder, as well as how effective the attempt was in achieving the stated goal. The most frequently endorsed reasons for these acts were: “to stop bad feelings”, “to punish myself”, “to relieve feelings of aloneness, emptiness or isolation”, “to obtain relief from a terrible state of mind”, and “to stop feeling so very sad”. When asked how effective the parasuicide attempt was in solving an endorsed problem, the attempt was rated as most effective for the following: “to punish myself”, “to prove to myself that things really were bad so it was ok to feel as bad as I did”, “to gain admission into a hospital or treatment program”, “to communicate with others and let others know how desperate I was”, and “to distract myself from other problems”. Thus, it is important for clinicians to recognize that there are varied reasons that these individuals engage in suicide attempts and other parasuicidal behavior. Even more importantly, clinicians must realize that it is difficult to eliminate a behavior (e.g., repeated suicide attempts) when the behavior is effective, albeit maladaptive. Indeed, these preliminary data suggest that this life-threatening behavior "works" in a number of ways that likely serve to reinforce the behavior. Therefore, much of the work among those with eating disorders who engage in parasuicidal behavior will be to find an alternative way to solve or better cope with these conflicts and problems.

Conclusions

In summary, mortality is substantially increased among people suffering from anorexia nervosa. The second leading cause of death among these individuals is suicide. Those who engage in purging appear to be at particularly increased risk for suicidal behavior. Those with anorexia nervosa have increased mortality compared to those with bulimia nervosa. However, many individuals with eating disorders who engage in other parasuicidal behavior such as intentional self-injury, do indeed have diagnoses of bulimia nervosa and again, almost always exhibit purging symptomatology.

Several predictors of suicidality in an eating disordered population, in addition to purging, have been identified. For those with anorexia nervosa, these risk factors include longer duration of illness, as well as presence and severity of substance abuse. Likewise among those with bulimia nervosa, a drug use disorder predicts suicide attempts, as does the use of laxatives. Additional identified predictors for those with bulimia nervosa include high levels of anger and abusive or otherwise traumatic childhoods. Importantly, the use of unhealthy weight control behaviors during adolescence, such as diet pill use or vomiting, predicts suicide attempts among young women years later.

Those individuals with eating disorders who have a history of suicidality are more likely than those with eating disorders but no suicide history to have experienced purging, co-morbid substance use disorders, anxiety disorders, and a history of childhood and/or sexual abuse. A subset of these individuals are classified as "multi-impulsive", as they exhibit a variety of additional impulsive behaviors such as shoplifting or sexual promiscuity and are more likely to have borderline personality pathology.

The most important thing for a clinician to keep in mind when working with an eating disordered population is the very real risk of suicide. This is the case particularly among patients with anorexia nervosa and even more so among those with a chronic course of illness that includes a past history of anorexia nervosa where there is a somewhat different current eating pathology presentation. In addition, those with bulimia nervosa who engage in repeated parasuicidal acts are at increased risk of death, as intentional self-injury may be fatal even when that was not the person's explicit intention. Therefore, a thorough suicide assessment must be conducted not just at the time of initial assessment, but as an ongoing part of treatment. For those patients for whom parasuicide is a chronic problem, the clinician must work collaboratively to determine the function it is serving and then develop alternative skills and coping strategies to replace this dangerous and maladaptive pattern of behavior.

Take home points

- Clinicians must always be aware of the significantly increased risk of suicide among individuals with EDs, particularly in the case of AN.
- In ED patients there is a need to conduct an especially careful current and ongoing assessment of the nature of any suicidality, degree of lethality and intention to die, particularly if any one or more of the following is true about the patient:
- has a current ED other than anorexia nervosa but has a past history of anorexia nervosa
- has anorexia nervosa with a long duration of illness
- engages in significant alcohol use after an acute period of anorexia nervosa
- engages in purging
- has bulimia nervosa plus any one or more of the following: abuses laxatives, a comorbid drug use disorder, high levels of anger, an abusive or traumatic childhood, or repeated past parasuicidal behavior.
- For those patients with EDs demonstrating chronic suicidal behavior, it is important to recognize that such behavior can serve a variety of different functions, which may differ markedly across individuals.
- Therefore, the clinician must conduct a detailed functional analysis of this behavior in order to identify all of the factors that are reinforcing its continuance, so that an intervention plan can be designed to interrupt the reinforcing cycle.

References

1. Vitousek K, Watson S, Wilson GT. Enhancing motivation for change in treatment resistant eating disorders. Clin Psychol Rev. 1998;18:391–420.
2. Sullivan PF. Mortality in anorexia nervosa. Am J Psychiatry. 1995;152:1073–4.
3. Crisp A, et al. Death, survival and recovery in anorexia nervosa: a thirty five year study. Eur Eat Disord Rev. 2006;14:168–75.
4. Pompili M, Mancinelli I, Girardi P, Ruberto A, Tatarelli R. Suicide in anorexia nervosa: a meta-analysis. Int J Eat Disord. 2004;36:99–103.
5. Kramer MS. Clinical epidemiology and biostatistics: a primer for clinical investigators and decision-makers. Berlin: Springer; 1988.
6. Corcos M, Taieb O, Benoit-Lamy S, Paterniti S, Jeammet P, Flament MF. Suicide attempts in women with bulimia nervosa: frequency and characteristics. Acta Psychiatr Scand. 2002;106:381–6.
7. Fichter MM, Quadflieg N, Hedlund S. Long-term course of binge eating disorder and bulimia nervosa: relevance for nosology and diagnostic criteria. Int J Eat Disord. 2008;41:577–86.

8. Norring CE, Sohlber SS. Outcome, recovery, relapse and mortality across six years in patients with clinical eating disorders. Acta Psychiatr Scand. 1993;87:437–44.
9. Deter HC, Herzog W. Anorexia nervosa in a long-term perspective: results of the Heidelberg-Mannheim Study. Psychosom Med. 1994;56:20–7.
10. Eckert ED, Halmi KA, Marchi P, Grove W, Crosby R. Ten-year follow-up of anorexia nervosa: clinical course and outcome. Psychol Med. 1995;25:143–56.
11. Keel PK, Dorer DJ, Eddy KT, Franko D, Charlatan DL, Herzog DB. Predictors of mortality in eating disorders. Arch Gen Psychiatry. 2003;60:179–83.
12. Su JC, Birmingham CL. Mortality in a cohort of eating disorder patients. 7th annual eating disorder research society meeting. Albuquerque: NM; 2001.
13. Lee S, Chan YY, Hsu LK. The intermediate-term outcome of Chinese patients with anorexia nervosa in Hong Kong. Am J Psychiatry. 2003;160:967–72.
14. Lowe B, Zipped S, Buchholz C, DuPont Y, Reaps DL, Herzog W. Long term outcome of anorexia nervosa in a prospective 21-year follow-up study. Psychol Med. 2001;31:881–90.
15. Herzog DB, Greenwood DN, Dorer DJ, Flores AT, Eke lad ER, Richards A, et al. Mortality in eating disorders: a descriptive study. Int J Eat Disord. 2000;28:20–6.
16. Jorgenson J. The epidemiology of eating disorders in Fyn County, Denmark, 1977–1986. Acta Psychiatr Scand. 1992;85:30–4.
17. Moller-Madsen SM, Nystrup J, Nielson S. Mortality of anorexia nervosa in Denmark 1970–1987. Ugeskr Laeger. 1998;160:5509–13.
18. Pagsberg AK, Wang AR. Epidemiology of anorexia nervosa and bulimia nervosa in Bornholm County, Denmark, 1970–1989. Acta Psychiatr Scand. 1994;90:259–65.
19. Emborg C. Mortality and causes of death in patients with eating disorders in Denmark 1970–1993. Ugeskr Laeger. 2001;163:3476–80.
20. Patton GC. Mortality in eating disorders. Psychol Med. 1988;18:947–51.
21. Toltrup K, Brinch M, Isager T. Long term outcome of 151 cases of anorexia nervosa. The Copenhagen anorexia nervosa follow-up study. Acta Psychiatr Scand. 1985;71:308–87.
22. Crisp AH, Callender JS, Halek C, Hsu LK. Long-term mortality in anorexia nervosa. A 20-year follow-up of the St. George's and Aberdeen cohorts. Br J Psychiatry. 1992;161:104–7.
23. Theander S. Anorexia nervosa: a psychiatric investigation of 94 female patients. Acta Psychiatr Scand Suppl. 1970;214:1–194.
24. Korndofer SR, Lucas AR, Suman VJ, Crowson CS, Krahn LE, Melton LJ 3rd. Long-term survival of patients with anorexia nervosa: a population-based study in Rochester, Minn. Mayo Clin Proc 2003;78:278–84.
25. Birmingham C, Su J, Hlysnky J, Goldner E, Gao M. The mortality rate from anorexia nervosa. Int J Eat Disord. 2005;38:1–4.
26. Steinhausen HC. Outcome of eating disorders. Child Adolesc Psychiatr Clin N Am. 2009;18:225–42.
27. Armson S. Stigmatization and suicide. In: Crisp AH, editor. Every family in the land. London: Royal Society of Medicine Press; 2004. p. 100–4.
28. Kreipe RE, Churchill BH, Strauss J. Long-term outcome of adolescents with anorexia nervosa. Am J Dis Child. 1989;143:1322–7.
29. Bulik CM, Thornton L, Pinheiro AP, Plotnicov K, Klump KL, Brandt H, et al. Suicide attempts in anorexia nervosa. Psychosom Med. 2008;70:378–83.
30. Linehan MM. Cognitive behavioral treatment of borderline personality disorder. New York: Guilford Press; 1993.
31. Favaro A, Santonastaso P. Purging behaviors, suicide attempts, and psychiatric symptoms in 398 eating disordered subjects. Int J Eat Disord. 1996;20:99–103.
32. Favaro A, Santonastaso P. Suicidality in eating disorders: clinical and psychological correlates. Acta Psychiatr Scand. 1997;95:508–14.
33. Favaro A, Santonastaso P. Impulsive and compulsive self-injurious behavior in bulimia nervosa: prevalence and psychological correlates. J Nerv Ment Dis. 1998;186:157–65.

34. Vandereycken W, Pierloot R. The significance of subclassification in anorexia nervosa: a comparative study of clinical features in 141 patients. Psychol Med. 1983;13:543–9.
35. Franko DL, Keel PK. Suicidality in eating disorders: occurrence, correlates, and clinical implications. Clin Psychol Rev. 2006;26:769–82.
36. Favaro A, Ferrara S, Santonastaso P. Self-injurious behavior in a community sample of young women: relationship with childhood abuse and other types of self damaging behaviors. J Clin Psychiatry. 2007;68:122–31.
37. Franko DL, Keel PK, Dorer DJ, Blais MA, Delinsky SS, Eddy KT, et al. What predicts suicide attempts in women with eating disorders? Psychol Med. 2004;34:843–53.
38. Bulik CM, Sullivan PF, Joyce PR. Temperament, character and suicide attempts in anorexia nervosa, bulimia nervosa and major depression. Acta Psychiatr Scand. 1999;100:27–32.
39. Nickel MK, Simek M, Lojewski N, Muehlbacher M, Fartacek R, Kettler C, et al. Familial and sociopsychopathological risk factors for suicide attempt in bulimic and in depressed women: prospective study. Int J Eat Disord. 2006;39:410–7.
40. Crow S, Eisenberg ME, Story M, Neumark-Sztainer D. Are body dissatisfaction, eating disturbance, and body mass index predictors of suicidal behavior in adolescents? A longitudinal study. J Consult Clin Psychol. 2008;76:887–92.
41. Milos G, Spindler A, Hepp U, Schnyder U. Suicide attempts and suicidal ideation: links with psychiatric comorbidity in eating disorder subjects. Gen Hosp Psychiatry. 2004;26:129–35.
42. Stein D, Lilenfeld LRR, Wildman PC, Marcus MD. Attempted suicide and self-injury in patients diagnosed with eating disorders. Compr Psychiatry. 2004;45:447–51.
43. Yamaguchi N, Kobayashi J, Tachikawa H, Sato S, Hori M, Suzuki T, et al. Parental representation in eating disorder patients with suicide. J Psychosom Res. 2000;49:131–6.
44. Lacey JH. Self-damaging and addictive behavior in bulimia nervosa: a catchment area study. Br J Psychiatry. 1993;163:190–4.
45. Fichter MM, Quadflieg N, Rief W. Course of multi-impulsive bulimia. Psychol Med. 1994;24:591–604.
46. Vitousek K, Manke F. Personality variables and disorders in anorexia nervosa and bulimia nervosa. J Abnorm Psychol. 1994;103:137–47.
47. Favaro A, Santonastaso P, Monteleone P, Bellodi L, Mauri M, Rotondo A, et al. Self-injurious behavior and attempted suicide in purging bulimia nervosa: associations with psychiatric comorbidity. J Affect Disord. 2008;20:99–103.
48. Wildman P, Lilenfeld LRR, Marcus MD. Axis I comorbidity onset and parasuicide in women with eating disorders. Int J Eat Disord. 2004;35:190–7.
49. Lucas AR, Beard CM, O'Fallon WM, Kurland LT. 50-year trends in the incidence of anorexia nervosa in Rochester, Minn.: a population based study. Am J Psychiatry. 1991;148:917–22.
50. Lilenfeld LRR, Levitt A, Stein D. The nature, function and efficacy of parasuicide among individuals with eating disorders. Forthcoming.

Chapter 6
Mothers with Eating Disorders: The Environmental Factors Affecting Eating-Related Emotional Difficulties in Their Offspring

Shiri Sadeh-Sharvit, Rachel Levy-Shiff, Anca Ram, Eitan Gur, Eynat Zubery, Evelyne Steiner and Yael Latzer

Abstract Eating disorders (EDs) have been explained by the Object Relations psychodynamic theory as resulting from maturation fears and separation difficulties in the origin family. The aim of this study was to understand from an Object Relations perspective, how mothers with EDs function with their toddlers, particularly with regard to disordered eating-related behavior. Twenty-nine dyads of mothers with EDs who had toddlers participated in a semi-structured interview, by which the environmental mechanisms of feeding, eating and emotional transactions were uncovered. The interviews revealed that some of the early needs of the mothers with EDs, that were unmet by their own parents, along with exaggerated anxiety about their children's eating and weight were associated with maternal accounts of EDs contents and practices, markedly with regard to daughters. The mothers' internal world was found to influence maternal practice in inadequate feeding of their toddlers. The findings imply that children of mothers with EDs should be viewed as potentially the next generation to express emotional difficulties through disrupted eating and body image.

S. Sadeh-Sharvit · R. Levy-Shiff
Department of Psychology, Bar Ilan University, Ramat Gan, Israel

S. Sadeh-Sharvit (✉) · E. Zubery · E. Steiner
Eating Disorders Treatment and Research Center, Hanotrim (Davidson) Clinic, Raanana, Shalvata Mental Health Center, Raanana, Israel
e-mail: shiri.sharvit@gmail.com

A. Ram
Children Ward, Beer Yaakov-Ness Ziona Mental Health Center, Ness Ziona, Israel

E. Gur
Eating Disorders Department, Sheba Medical Center, Tel Hashomer, Ramat Gan, Israel

Y. Latzer
Faculty of Social Welfare and Health Science, Haifa University, Haifa, Israel

Y. Latzer
Eating Disorders Institute, Psychiatry Division, Rambam Medical Center, Haifa, Israel

Y. Latzer and D. Stein (eds.), *Bio-Psycho-Social Contributions to Understanding Eating Disorders*, DOI 10.1007/978-3-319-32742-6_6

Introduction

Object Relations conceptualization of the development of eating disorders placed their psychological onset in early childhood and specifically in the nature of the caretakers-child relationship. Therefore, psychodynamic theories as well as therapeutic interventions focused on female adolescents and young female adults [1–4].[1] Recently, the continuation of EDs along the life cycle has received increasing attention. Therapists and researchers realize that adult women with EDs suffer from similar enduring symptoms while coping with different developmental challenges in their lives, such as building a family [5]. Highly intriguing is the question, how do disrupted parent-child relations in the origin family influence the maternal functioning of the mothers with EDs with their own children? In this chapter we will present a study which investigated this question from a psychodynamic object-relations perspective.

Perseverance of EDs Symptoms Throughout Adult Life

Longitudinal studies found that EDs are characterized by a long duration and a high relapse rate, even following long periods of remission [6]. Other studies revealed that some personality traits of women with EDs remained stable after the remission of symptoms. For instance, women with a past—but not current—ED were found to display more anxiety, depression, and obsessive symptoms, along with rigid thinking, narrowed emotional expression, excessive attempts to control themselves and their drives, and low interpersonal spontaneity [7–9].

Approximately half of the women with EDs in the age range of 20–45 are involved in a spousal relationship [10]; some build a family. The fertility of women with EDs is quite low; however, some successfully conceive, even with a low BMI and irregular menstrual cycles, partly thanks to fertility treatments [11–13]. Many postpartum mothers with EDs are at a high risk of developing psychiatric problems, such as postpartum depression and symptomatic deterioration [14, 15].

Parental Functioning of Mothers with EDs

The existing research on mothers with EDs is limited, especially considering the high risk potential of transmission of the disorder in families. The existing accumulative evidence is extremely disturbing; it suggests that mothers with EDs are overly preoccupied with their children's eating and thinness. For instance,

[1] The present study focuses on EDs among women who are also mothers. Consequently, the feminine gender is used throughout this chapter.

researchers have found that the more severe the maternal ED, the more anxious the mothers are in regard to the child's appearance, and their interaction with the child during feeding times is more intrusive [16–18]. Moreover, it was revealed that children of mothers with EDs exhibit more psychiatric problems, such as EDs, obsessive compulsive disorder (OCD), oppositional disorder, and enuresis [19–22].

Parental psychiatric disorders may significantly influence child rearing practices, and be a risk factor for the development of mental disorders among children, beyond the genetic contribution [23–27]. An ED may be one of the most influential maternal illnesses on young children due to the fact that eating is a central daily routine in mother-child interaction and this maternal mental disorder may be more influential on the child. Hence it was hypothesized that a maternal ED may compromise maternal functioning. The current study also sought to examine the intrapersonal mechanisms that may be involved in maternal functioning, and understand them in light of an object relations explanation for eating disorder development.

Data Collection

Fifty-eight dyads of mothers and toddlers participated in the research (a total of 116 participants): 29 dyads of mothers with EDs and their children and 29 mothers in a control group. The children's ages ranged from 18 to 36 months. Dyads of mothers and children in the control group were matched to the research group in regard to the mother's age and education and the child's gender, age, and birth order. The average age of the mothers in the EDs group was 31, and 33 (SDs were 4.2 and 4.6, respectively) in the control group ($t = -1.79$ ns). The average age of the toddlers in the research groups was 32.5 ($SD = 7.2$) and 30.6 ($SD = 7.3$) months, respectively ($t = 1.05$ ns). 65 % of the children were girls.

Mothers in the EDs group were recruited from three psychiatric treatment units in Israel, and were diagnosed before participating in the study as suffering from anorexia nervosa (AN), bulimia nervosa (BN) or eating disorder not otherwise specified (EDNOS). Seventeen mothers were treated in EDs outpatient treatment at the time of the study, and none were hospitalized at the time. 27 of 29 mothers (93 %) reported having ED symptoms at the time of the study.

Data was collected using self-report measures of current maternal ED and comorbid symptoms, maternal stress, and support resources. Each child underwent a psychodevelopmental evaluation, and the home milieu was assessed as well. Mother-child interactions were video-recorded during a semi-structured situation and were later coded by skilled judges, blind to group membership. Detailed descriptions of the tools and quantitative findings are provided in the original report [28].

Additionally, each mother with an ED participated in a semi-structured interview developed and carried out by the chapter's first author. The interviews lasted approximately 60 min, and aimed at revealing the participants' subjective experience of motherhood and the effects of their ED on their maternal functioning.

The interview focused on four key issues: (A) past and current ED symptoms, (B) transition to motherhood, (C) present maternal functioning and the mother-child relationship, and (D) the spousal relationship and her partner's attitude toward her ED. Interpretation of the interview was performed by the first author with content analysis. The central categories and explanations that emerged independently from the interviews were sorted into central themes [29].

Main Quantitative Results

Paramount quantitative findings are delineated hereinafter. Full descriptions of the results can be found in an earlier report [28]. Consistent significant differences were found between mothers with EDs and their children in comparison to the dyads in the control group, in all study variables, except for maternal body mass index (BMI), in which no significant difference was found. Findings suggest that mothers with EDs exhibit significantly higher psychopathological symptoms of eating and comorbid disorders. Mothers with EDs also displayed problematic maternal functioning: they were significantly more likely to report high maternal stress and more negative emotions toward their children. In addition, mothers with EDs tended to organize the home surroundings to meet the child's developmental needs less than mothers without EDs. Spousal and social support buffered the negative effect of the mother's eating disorder on her maternal functioning and child outcome.

The children of mothers with EDs received lower scores on the mental, psychomotor, and socio-emotional developmental scales. These children also showed more symptoms and problems, such as anxiety/depression and somatization. Mother-child interactions analysis revealed that mothers with EDs demonstrated more intrusiveness, lower emotional responsiveness, and less complex cognitive mediation. The mother-child interactions in the EDs group were characterized by less cooperation, less desire for closeness, and less verbal communication and more emotional lability.

Main Themes Emerged from the Interviews with Mothers with EDs

Five central content categories were found in the interviews with the mothers with EDs. The following themes were analyzed according to the object relations conceptualization of EDs, which is interweaved throughout the following quotes.[2]

[2]The mothers' quotations are graphically differentiated with a different font and text indentation. Short quotes of up to three sentences are presented in the text in a different font.

Deficiency in Libidinal Resources to Invest in the Child

The etiology of EDs is complex and involves interaction of genetic, biologic, psychological, and socio-cultural factors [30, 31]. According to the object relations school, a conflictual parent-child relationship creates sensitivity for EDs among some female adolescents. During the course of development, in some of the families the parents find it difficult to allow the girl to separate from them psychologically and develop an autonomous self. This results in boundary confusion between the girl and her parents, who often respond to their child in regard to their own needs, as a narcissistic extension of themselves. Such symbiosis endorses a highly dependent relationship and diminishes the girl's ability to build a cohesive, independent, and regulated self [32]. During childhood, the symbiotic relationship between the girl and her parents is experienced as satisfactory for both sides. However, in adolescence, the developmental demands for maturation and separation, along with the increasing attention to the body, femininity, and sexuality, disquiet the fragmental internal and interpersonal homeostasis. The over-dependent girl develops into an adolescent who marvels at self-control and self-punishment and expresses her emotions, needs, and internal conflicts through her body and, more concretely, via the function of feeding and eating [1, 33].

According to this conceptualization, an ED is viewed as a coping mechanism that protects the patient from her fear of psychological separation from the origin family [30, 32]. Therefore, part of the self of mothers with EDs may be preoccupied with pre-oedipal conflicts with the parental objects [2, 34], while other self parts demand to perform psychosocial appropriate functioning, such as taking care of the new family. This picture becomes more complex particularly when dealing with mothers of toddlers, on whom the current research focused. Interviews with mothers with EDs revealed that they tended to describe themselves as moving up and down on a continuum between libidinal investment in adult functioning as mothers, spouses, and career women and regression into a childlike yearning for the fulfillment of early needs they perceived as unmet. Mothers expressed difficulties in being the caretakers of their toddlers, especially in their children's dependence in them. One mother articulated it well:

> I'm still a little girl that seeks Mommy's love. Someone has to feed me and take care of me… Until I learn to take care of myself, cook, eat, be responsible for myself, and stop waiting that someone else will cook for me and feed me and think for me and take care of me, until I stop this thing, it will be impossible for me to take care of others, who are in this case my son and daughter.

The interviews shed light on mothers with EDs' limited libidinal resources to invest in themselves, even more so in their children. An unconscious fear emerged: that fulfillment of their children's needs would leave the mothers' psychological resources depleted. Hence, mothers with EDs find it difficult to invest emotionally in their children and serve as a stable source for mirroring and containment. In other words, the mothers' deficiency of internal good and empowering objects—an inherent characteristic of EDs—disrupts the women's maternal functioning. In some families, this role confusion was intensified, with the child becoming a parental child with implicit responsibility for the mother's emotional well-being. For instance, one of the mothers said of her firstborn son, an older sibling of the child that participated in the study:

> He's a very special child, mature for his age. Maybe it [her ED] has made him like that. He's very introverted, shuts it all inside… When I'm in the bathroom, he knows I'm there, and he knows what I do there. You can't hide it. And he doesn't interrupt and doesn't call me [at these times]. I think he should receive from me much more than I can really give… He called me at night and said, 'Mommy, I pray you'll be healthy.' He didn't say what I have, but clearly he realizes.

Transgenerational Transmission of EDs

The interviews indicated a strong environmental effect of the maternal ED on the transactions she has with her children. The average age of the mothers in the research group was 31, while the average of the disorder onset was reported as 14. Hence, the mothers who participated in the study had been coping with an ED for 17 years on average before the transition to motherhood. Therefore, motherhood developed many years after an ED was embedded in the mother's personality and self-concept.

In the object relations formulation, EDs are associated with a struggle for separation and independence, which takes place in the eating domain and impairs the person's somatopsychological differentiation. Consequently, the boundaries between the attitude of mothers with EDs toward their own eating and body and toward these aspects in their children are blurred. Interviews suggest that mothers with EDs are very much concerned for their children's appearance and weight, and this is translated to a wish to control the child's caloric consumption. For example, mothers who recognized in their child a tendency to gain weight easily, or to enjoy eating, often experienced an emotional rejection of the child, as depicted in the following quote:

> It's OK when my kids eat a massive amount of food, as long as they're skinny. My third child is chubby, and this takes control of me; it scares me. I feel as if my illness takes over there. I feel I pass on my illness to him, whether I want to or not. I pay attention to what he eats, and comment on his speed, eating time, the amounts… At some stage, I tell him, 'That's it, you've eaten enough!' I try to teach him a little. I see a very big difficulty in my relationship with this child because he's more rotund. He's not fat, but my other children are skinny and very active, and they eat healthily. And him, I feel a less warm attitude toward this child, because he eats a lot and because he loves eating a lot of carbs. Because he enjoys food, you see a child who takes pleasure in every bite, and it simply tortures me. With my other children who eat the minimum they need, I sympathize much more. I feel that I identify much less with him, much less empathic to him. Watching him eat is extremely difficult for me. I mean, he eats, and I immediately translate each of his bites into tiny fat molecules in his body. And I immediately translate it into him not being popular and never having a girlfriend, and I've already attached homosexuality to him in my mind.

According to object relations theory, in the origin families of girls with EDs, the defense mechanism of projective identification, in which the person splits between good parts and bad unwanted parts of the self and projects the latter on others, is common [4, 35]. The parents project unwanted parts on the girl, who accepts and identifies with these parts. For example, this defense mechanism may be involved in the unconscious handling of intense needs and feelings, in the origin family [36]. When the girl becomes a mother herself, her children may turn into an object of splits and projections: the next generation preoccupied with issues of control and restraint and an internal world of persecutory internal objects [37].

The interviews also suggested the toddlers' preliminary awareness of their mothers' EDs symptoms. For example, one mother said, "I don't remember who of them asked me, 'Mommy, did you throw up?' or 'Do you vomit?,' so I responded, 'No,' or told them, 'Don't be nosy!'" Another interviewee recalled an episode from the preceding week: "The bathroom door was shut and they opened it, and Guy asked me, 'Mommy, you don't want to keep the food?'" These representative quotes suggest that in families in which the mother has an ED, the familial unconscious world is filled with implicit and indirect EDs themes. The toddlers, attentive to their parents as every child, may not only be aware of the maternal ED but also try and imitate it as part of the identification and internalization processes with the maternal object.

Difficulties in Toddlers' Actual Feeding

The intrapsychic worries of mothers with EDs and their implicit influence on the mother-child relationship have been presented. In addition, evidence of problems in actual maternal functioning was found in one sphere, feeding of the child. It was found that mothers with EDs exhibit feeding difficulties of their toddlers. The maternal anguish about her child becoming overweight in conjunction with food phobia and erroneous beliefs become joined in the child's body, which serves as the concrete realization of the mother's internal world. One mother describes well the boundary confusion between her feelings and thoughts regarding food, and feeding her child:

> Food is a very problematic issue between us. Again, he didn't suffer from it, but I did. I still tend to feed him sometimes, or do it when he's not aware of it, for instance while he is watching a movie. It's clear that no one really wants to eat, so I prefer to feed him when he is distracted. One of my greatest joys is when I put a plate in front of him, and he eats… [During the transition to solids] I was very nervous by the change in routine, introducing something new. My starting point is that it is clear that he wouldn't want to eat. I didn't think he could enjoy it. And it indeed was a self-fulfilling prophecy; he didn't want to eat fruits, for example. So we moved to Gerber's, and it was easier for me that it's already made and not something I have to prepare.

The immense anxiety these mothers experience in regard to their children's eating and bodies leads to active efforts to restrict the children's eating. Among these efforts, the following acts have been mentioned by mothers: avoidance of going to playgrounds in an attempt to prevent other people from feeding the child; placing children in a high chair even when it no longer fits their bodies but leaves them dependent on the feeding mother, who supervises the amounts of food eaten; postponing the transition to solids; and stopping the meal when the mother is afraid the child has eaten too much, despite of the child's continuing signals for hunger and interest in the food. Many mothers also have difficulties in offering varied meals that include all major food groups, as a consequence of their ED. The mother's conflicted attitude to eating may be internalized in a continuous process, and may become an inherent part of the mother-child relationship and the child's attitudes. One of the mothers with EDs described her daughter:

> I do see her thin [in the future]. Maybe thin because it would become part of her, or thin because it's a body structure, or thin because of the disorder [the maternal ED], I don't have a clue. I just see her skinny, at least the way she grows up now… Every time I sat next to her, she wouldn't eat. She got up in the middle [of the meal] and played with the food, so many problems. But when I wasn't around, she ate. She was disciplined and did eat. True, she doesn't eat much, but she does eat, something gets to her stomach. And when I'm around—nothing.

The interviews untangled that mothers with EDs' self-dysregulation of hunger and satiation disturbs child feeding as well. These mothers' perceptions of children's age-appropriate eating habits, food quantities, and variety are flawed. Some also obsessively regard each nutritional component separately and are uncertain how to integrate ingredients into a meal. It may be that, in this manner, mothers with EDs may potentially compromise the development of their children's self-awareness and self-regulation not only in the eating sphere but also in much broader aspects, such as emotional regulation and reflective functioning.

The aforementioned feeding interactions may affect children of mothers with EDs to distance themselves from their authentic bodily experience and understand their bodies differently, in a manner that fits the mother's needs [32]. These difficulties in toddlers' feeding create a risk not only for a transgenerational transmission of distorted body image and faulty eating patterns but also for reenactment of the premorbid intrapsychic foundation of EDs: The mother's incompatible reactions to the physical and emotional needs of the child might produce problems in the child's self-development, and especially influence low self-awareness and sense of control [38, 39].

Exaggerated Anxiety in Regard to Daughters' Eating and Body

The fears of mothers with EDs for their children's eating and body were found to be much more intense for their girls, who are at a heightened risk of suffering from EDs in the first place [40]. When mothers with EDs spoke of their daughters in comparison to their sons, they tended to express higher rates of anxiety as well as more negative evaluations of the daughter's feminine body and a stronger fear of her becoming fat. Mothers with EDs also reported more difficulties in feeding daughters and their daughters' independent eating. Keeping the object relations theory in mind, these mothers' difficulty in accepting their daughters as separate persons with their own appetite and body was uncovered. A mother of children of both sexes stated:

> I honestly don't know, if I were to choose for my girl, to be fat or have an eating disorder, I don't know what I would prefer. I feel very bad for thinking this, I think it makes me a bad mother… When I feed them both [her son and daughter], I give him a much larger portion than the one she receives. Him I feed when he doesn't eat well, and with her, I insist that no one else would feed her. She feeds herself, and the minute she doesn't want the food anymore, we take away her plate. Because if you push food into her mouth, she'd eat.

The interviews revealed that among mothers with EDs, the ED played a much more significant role in the mother-daughter relationship in comparison to these mothers' relationships with their sons. According to psychodynamic theories on normal feminine identity development, a mother-daughter dyad is different from a mother-son dyad in nature. The mother-daughter relationship tends to be characterized by more blurred psychological boundaries; mothers are more likely to experience their daughters as an extension and continuation of themselves, and girls experience themselves as less separated from their mothers [41]. This conceptualization explains why mothers with EDs tend to project more unwanted self-parts on their daughters, namely, their own eating and body shape concerns. Thus, the stronger closeness between mothers and daughters puts daughters of mothers with EDs at a heightened risk of internalization and learning by imitating the mothers' ED symptoms.

Moreover, our research found that the level of maternal anxiety and preoccupation in EDs themes in regard to daughters was higher for older daughters. It may be that the more apparent the separation potential, the more the detachment fears and EDs concerns merge with one another and increase the risk the daughter will also experience unhealthy attitudes toward her eating and body. Hence, the mother's increased anxiety about her daughter's body and maturation in general might undermine the needs of the daughter's developing self [32].

Motherhood as an Opportunity for Reparation and Reintegration

Motherhood arouses in women a strong urge for health, growth, and love, and maintains hope for further development and change [42]. The interviews revealed that mothers with EDs experienced motherhood as another stressor, but at the same time the child marked the possibility of reparation: a second chance for the mothers to express their "inner child," the healthy strengths inside them. According to object relations theory, the fundamental developmental task not fully accomplished in EDs is separation from the parental objects [43]. Motherhood offers another opportunity to displace the cathexis invested in the past to the new intimate relationship with the child [34].

For some mothers, the fear of transgenerational transmission of their ED led to partial remission of symptoms. For example, the following mother demonstrates the effort of symptom diminishment:

> I start worrying for my girl as well, because I've seen my dad like this. In a few years from now, she'll be all grown up, and I don't want her to see her mother binge at night. Until today, I haven't sought treatment, and I am predominantly interested in it now because of her… I've realized it [her ED] takes a whole lot of energy from me, and it's a pity as I need this energy. Don't know, it's a matter of growing up. It bugs me. How come I can't control my impulses? What kind of a thing is that?… Motherhood made me want more to take care of it. If I had become a mother a few years ago, then I would have turned to treatment earlier. I just went with the flow of it back then. You can live with it [her ED], and you don't die from it. But when you see that you need the energy, and you don't want your daughter to grow up just like you. You just can't push it aside. In a sense, it's good that Naomi was born.

Discussion

The overarching aim of this research was to study the psychological and maternal functioning of mothers with EDs and their children's development and adaptation. The current report focused on the psychodynamic perspective of object relations in understanding the transactions between mothers with EDs and their toddlers. Object relations approach, which originally elucidated the development of EDs among adolescent girls, was employed here to explain some aspects in the mother-child relationship. According to object relations theories, EDs are associated with boundary confusion between the girl and the parental objects, and intense separation anxiety. EDs express the girl's difficulties in individuation and maturation, which manifest in the eating and body domains and disrupt her somatopsychological functioning. Hence, in the face of adulthood challenges, the girl could regress to a childlike stance and may find it difficult to adaptively manage the new psycho-developmental and social tasks [1, 37, 43]. The contents of the interviews, along with the quantitative findings, suggest that the characterizing psychological conflicts that preoccupied the mothers' minds before conception persist to some extent, as a possibly inherent feature of maternal functioning and the mother-child relationship. In other words, the offspring of mothers with EDs are in high risk of becoming the next generation for psychological difficulties, in the eating domain as well as in other areas of development.

In the object relations formulation, mothers' with EDs lifelong conflict between rejection of their early needs and separation may potentially put their children at risk for receiving maternal treatment that is less compatible with the child's needs [44]. The maternal preoccupation with eating and body, shape and weight may load the child's inner world with ED concerns that may be viewed by these children as egosyntonic [45–47]. Moreover, feeding is the primal interaction in the mother-child relationship, through which early objects develop [48]. Therefore, the feeding difficulties reported along with normal imitation learning and identification processes make EDs a real and immediate problem for these children, which may develop simultaneously with the construction of the child's inner world. A mother-child relationship consists of symbiotic and separated elements at the same time [49]. Hence, children of mothers with EDs may experience, too, issues of symbiosis, intrusiveness, and separation-anxiety of the maternal object, and express them via the eating and body spheres. Given that maternal object internalization could be colored by an eating and body discourse, the child's attempts at separation might be exhibited by it as well.

Another critical finding in our research is that during the feeding interactions, mothers with EDs unconsciously reinforce the child to distance himself or herself from his or her authentic experience, at the soma level and in a more abstract realm. As a consequence of identifying with the mother's needs and preferences, children of mothers with EDs may deny or repress their internal phenomena. This process may result in disruption of recognition of inner states, including hunger and satiation cues, and in a diminished sense of self-control. This dynamic might characterize the matrix of the development of an ED among these toddlers [1, 4, 32, 33, 39]. Additionally, finding suggest that the daughters of mothers with EDs are at an increased risk of bonding with their mothers through a shared pursuit of thinness, control and denial of fundamental needs.

Undoubtedly, EDs include a strong genetic component, but they also run in families through environmental influences and a psychological transgenerational transmission [31, 50–52]. Evidence implies that maternal ED may significantly intensify the children's risk of struggling with an ED. Nevertheless, this study also demonstrated that the influence of the maternal ED on maternal functioning is not predestined. Motherhood brought about an opportunity for psychological reparation; mothers reported attempts to minimize their symptoms and not reenact with their children the parent-child relationship of their origin family.

The current research focused on the mother-child relationship in families in which the mother has a lifetime ED. Further research should expand the perspective to the parents-child tryad, and explore fathers' possible moderating role in the manifestation of the maternal ED in the child's life. Moreover, children of mothers with EDs should be viewed as children at increased risk for developmental and emotional problems. Future interventions focusing on supporting the maternal functioning of women with eating disorders could prove beneficial in terms of both mother and child outcomes. An evidence-based prevention-intervention program for families in which the mother has an ED has been developed by three of the authors (SSS, EZ, and ES), and is being carried out and evaluated, in an attempt to enhance the adaptive functioning of these families.

Take home points

- Maternal eating disorder may compromise maternal functioning.
- Toddlers of mothers with EDs are nurtured in a context of high maternal distress and decreased availability of emotional resources to invest in the child.
- Normal mother-child conflicts are aggregated in the food and eating domains and a transgenerational transmission of eating problems may develop within the new family.
- Interventions with children of mothers with EDs should include a detailed report of the eating practices of all family members.
- Increased paternal involvement and a more structured daily routine may mitigate the influence of maternal ED on the distress and disordered eating of young children.

References

1. Bruch H. Eating disorders: obesity, anorexia nervosa and the person within. London: Routledge Kegan Paul; 1973.
2. Selvini-Palazzoli M. Self starvation. New York, NY: Aronson; 1974.
3. Sours JA. Starving to death in a sea of objects. New York, NY: Aronson; 1980.
4. Masterson JF. Primary anorexia nervosa in the borderline adolescent: An object-relations view. In: Hartocollis P, editor. Borderline personality disorders: The concept, the syndrome, the patient. New York, NY: International Universities Press; 1977. p. 475–94.
5. Stein A, Woolley H, McPherson K. Conflict between mothers with eating disorders and their infants during mealtimes. Br J Psychiatry. 1999;175:455–61.
6. Herzog DB, Dorer DJ, Keel PK, Selwyn SE, Ekeblad ER, Flores A, et al. Recovery and relapse in anorexia and bulimia nervosa: A 7.5-year follow-up study. J Am Acad Child Adolesc Psychiatry. 1999;38:829–37.
7. Le Grange D, Binford RB, Peterson CB, Crow SJ, Crosby RD, Klein MH, et al. DSM-IV threshold versus subthreshold bulimia nervosa. Int J Eat Disord. 2006;39(6):462–7.
8. Kaye WH, Klump KL, Frank GKW, Strober M. Anorexia and bulimia nervosa. Annu Rev Med. 2000;51:299–313.
9. Wagner A, Barbarich-Marsteller NC, Frank GK, Bailer UF, Wonderlich SA, Crosby RD, et al. Personality traits after recovery from eating disorders: Do subtypes differ? Int J Eat Disord. 2006;39(4):276–84.
10. Wiederman MW, Pryor TA. Comparison of ever-married and never-married women with anorexia nervosa or bulimia nervosa. Int J Eat Disord. 1997;22(4):395–401.
11. Stewart DE, Robinson GE, Goldbloom DS, Wright C. Infertility and eating disorders. Am J Obstet Gynecol. 1990;163:1196–9.
12. Bonne OB, Rubinoff B, Berry EM. Delayed detection of pregnancy in patients with Anorexia Nervosa: Two case reports. Int J Eat Disord. 1996;20(4):423–5.
13. Mazzeo SE, Zucker NL, Gerke CK, Mitchell K, Bulik CM. Parenting concerns of women with histories of eating disorders. Int J Eat Disord. 2005;35:S77–9.
14. Franko DL, Blais MA, Becker AE, Selwyn-Delinsky S, Greenwood DN, Flores AT, et al. Pregnancy complications and neonatal outcomes in women with eating disorders. Am J Psychiatry. 2001;158:1461–6.
15. Morgan JF, Lacey JH, Sedgwick PM. Impact of pregnancy on bulimia nervosa. Br J Psychiatry. 1999;174:135–40.

16. Stein A, Murray L, Cooper P, Fairburn CG. Infant growth in the context of maternal eating disorders and maternal depression: A comparative study. Psychol Med. 1996;26:569–74.
17. Russell GFM, Treasure J, Eisler I. Mothers with anorexia nervosa who underfeed their children: Their recognition and management. Psychol Med. 1998;28:93–108.
18. Waugh E, Bulik CM. Offspring of women with eating disorders. Int J Eat Disord. 1999;25:123–33.
19. Hodes M, Timimi S, Robinson P. Children of mothers with eating disorders: A preliminary study. Eur Eat Disord Rev. 1997;5(1):11–24.
20. Stein A, Woolley H, Cooper SD, Fairburn CG. An observational study of mothers with eating disorders and their infants. J Psychoanal Psychiatry. 1994;35(4):733–48.
21. Stein A, Woolley H, Cooper S, Winterbottom J, Fairburn CG, Cortina-Borja M. Eating habits and attitudes among 10-year-old children of mothers with eating disorders: Longitudinal study. Br J Psychiatry. 2006;189:324–9.
22. Stein A, Woolley H, Senior R, Hertzmann L, Lovel M, Lee J, Cooper S, et al. Treating disturbances in the relationship between mothers with bulimic eating disorders and their infants: A randomized, controlled trial of video feedback. Am J Psychiatry. 2006;163:899–906.
23. Boyle MH, Pickles A. Maternal depressive symptoms and ratings of emotional disorder symptoms in children and adolescents. J Child Psychol Psychiatry. 1997;38:981–92.
24. Cassidy B, Zoccolillo M, Hughes S. Psychopathology in adolescent mothers and its effects on mother-infant interactions: A pilot study. Can J Psychiatry. 1996;41:379–84.
25. Marshall T, Jones DPH, Ramchandani PG, Stein A, Bass C. Intergenerational transmission of health beliefs in somatoform disorders. Br J Psychiatry. 2007;191(4):449–50.
26. Turner SM, Beidel DC, Epstein LH. Vulnerability and risk for anxiety disorders. J Anxiety Disord. 1991;5(2):151–66.
27. Weinberg MK, Tronick EZ. The impact of maternal psychiatric illness on infant development. J Clin Psychiatry. 1998;59(Suppl. 2):53–61.
28. Sadeh-Sharvit S. Mothers with eating disorders: Maternal functioning, child development and behavior [PhD thesis]. Ramat Gan: Bar-Ilan University, Psychology Department; 2008.
29. Strauss AL, Corbin JM. Basics of qualitative research: Grounded theory procedures and techniques. Newbury Park, CA: Sage Publications; 1990.
30. Becker AE, Grinspoon SK, Klibansky A, Herzog DB. Current concepts: Eating disorders. N Engl J Med. 1999;340(14):1092–8.
31. Bulik CM. Exploring the gene-environment nexus in eating disorders. J Psychiatry Neurosci. 2005;30(5):335–9.
32. Bruch H. The golden cage: The Enigma of Anorexia Nervosa. Cambridge, MA: Harvard University Press; 1978.
33. Boris HR. On the treatment of anorexia nervosa. Int J Psychoanal. 1984;65:435–42.
34. Fischer N. Anorexia Nervosa and unresolved rapprochement conflicts: a case study. Int J Psychoanal. 1989;70:41–54.
35. Klein M. Notes on some schizoid mechanisms. Int J Psychoanal. 1946;27:99–110.
36. Humphrey LL. Object relations and the family system: An integrative approach to understanding and treating eating disorders. In: Johnson C, editor. Psychodynamic Treatment of Anorexia Nervosa and Bulimia. New York, NY: Guilford Press; 1991. p. 321–53.
37. Lane RC. Anorexia, masochism, self-mutilation, and autoerotism: The spider mother. Psychoanal Rev. 2002;89(1):101–23.
38. Boris HR. The problem of anorexia nervosa. Int J Psychoanal. 1984;65:315–22.
39. Johnson C. Treatment of eating-disordered patients with borderline and false-self/narcissistic disorders. In: Johnson C, editor. Psychodynamic Treatment of Anorexia Nervosa and Bulimia. New York, NY: Guilford Press; 1991. p. 165–93.
40. American Psychiatric Association. Diagnostic and statistical manual of mental disorders. 4th ed. Washington, DC: APA; 1994.
41. Chodorow N. The reproduction of mothering. CA: University of California Press; 1978.

42. Winnicott DW. Through pediatrics to psycho-analysis. London: Hogarth Press; 1956. Primary maternal preoccupation; p. 300–5.
43. Sours JA. The anorexia nervosa syndrome. Int J Psychoanal. 1974;55(4):567–76.
44. Winnicott DW. The maturational process and the facilitating environment. New York, NY: International Universities Press; 1965.
45. Danieli Y. Families of survivors of the Nazi Holocaust: some short and long term effects. In: Spielberger CD, Sarason IG, Milgram NA, editors. Stress and Anxiety. Vol. 8. Washington, DC: Hemisphere; 1982. p. 405–19.
46. Rakoff V, Sigal JJ, Epstien NB, Nathan B. Working through in joint family therapy. Am J Psychother. 1967;21:782–90.
47. Schwartz S, Dohrenwend BP, Levav I. Nongenetic familial transmission of psychiatric disorders? Evidence from children of Holocaust survivors. J Health Soc Behav. 1994;35 (4):385–402.
48. Klein M. A contribution to the psychogenesis of manic-depressive states. Int J Psychoanal. 1935;16:145–74.
49. Mahler MS. On the three subphases of the separation individuation process. Int J Psychoanal. 1972;53:333–8.
50. Coulthard H, Blissett J, Harris G. The relationship between parental eating problems and children's feeding behavior: a selective review of the literature. Eat Behav. 2004;5(2):103–15.
51. Hinney A, Friedel S, Remschmidt H, Hebebrand J. Genetic risk factors in eating disorders. Am J Pharmacogenomics. 2004;4(4):209–23.
52. Klump KL, Wonderlich S, Lehoux P, Lilenfeld LR, Bulik CM. Does environment matter? A review of nonshared environment and eating disorders. Int J Eat Disord. 2002;31(2):118–35.

Chapter 7
Giving 'Til It Hurts': Eating Disorders and Pathological Altruism

R. Bachner-Melman and B. Oakley

Abstract When the willingness to place another's perceived needs above one's own in a way that causes self-harm, the normally positive and necessary characteristic of altruism can become unhealthy. "Pathological altruism" has been the focus of a recent surge of theoretical, philosophical, clinical and empirical interest. This chapter explores its relevance to individuals suffering from eating disorders, who can be viewed as prototypical pathological altruists. Both genetic and environmental factors contribute to a poorly defined sense of self and the resulting adaptation to external expectations and devotion to others' needs. A façade of self-sufficiency, all too often misinterpreted as a sign of health, belies the natural need to receive from others. A fear of losing relationships, a need for approval, and conscious or unconscious anger at self-sacrifice lend a flavor of martyrdom to the act of giving. The endorsement of the thin beauty ideal underlying eating disorders may be seen as a form of pathological altruism, since the biological need to eat is sacrificed to the "needs" or dictates of society concerning body shape. Anecdotal, theoretical, clinical and empirical support for pathological altruism in eating disordered patients is presented, as well as implications for treatment, recovery and prevention.

R. Bachner-Melman
Social and Community Sciences, Ruppin Academic Center,
40250 Emek Hefer, Israel

R. Bachner-Melman (✉)
Psychology Department, Hebrew University of Jerusalem,
91905 Jerusalem, Israel
e-mail: rachel.bachner@mail.huji.ac.il

B. Oakley
School of Engineering and Computer Science, Oakland University,
Rochester 48306, USA

Y. Latzer and D. Stein (eds.), *Bio-Psycho-Social Contributions to Understanding Eating Disorders*, DOI 10.1007/978-3-319-32742-6_7

Pathological Altruism

Surely There Couldn't *Be Anything Wrong with Altruism?*

After all, over the past century thousands of articles and books on altruism have pointed out that caring for others is central to all human social structures. The study of altruism has recently gained momentum as neuroscience has revealed the role of genetics and neurophysiology in our feelings of compassion and empathy [1]. It appears we are hardwired to care for others. And if most of us derive a sense of competence, pleasure and self-worth from being kind, helpful and generous towards others, how could altruism be pathological?

Many researchers are so invested in the benefits of altruism that they frown on studies emphasizing its potential pitfalls. Western societies have become so focused on its benefits that its flip side has been virtually ignored. The first known reference to "pathological altruism" in the professional literature is in a paper by Seelig and Rosof written in 2001: "Normal and Pathological Altruism", which explores the concept from a psychoanalytic perspective [2]. The concept of misplaced, harmful altruism has recently been consolidated in a volume entitled *Pathological Altruism* [3], which provides a new and helpful framework for understanding detrimental social processes ranging from pet hoarding, to the *DSM-5's* dependent personality disorder, to misspent foreign aid that supports tyrannical dictatorships, and indeed, to genocide itself.

For the purposes of this chapter, pathological altruism can be defined as "the willingness of a person to irrationally place another's perceived needs above his or her own in a way that causes self-harm" [4, 5]. The major motivations for giving in healthy altruism are openness to new experiences and a desire for personal growth [6]. In contrast, the major motivation in pathological altruism is to enhance a sense of self-worth via significant self-sacrifice and self-deprivation [2]. The point at which giving becomes unhealthy is difficult to define.

Codependency is one example of pathological altruism, in which a person inadvertently supports another's dysfunctional behavior, often at a cost in health and lifestyle to the codependent. This phenomenon has received extraordinary popular interest over the past decades, with over four million copies of Melodie Beatty's *Codependent No More* sold since its publication in 1986. Yet, as psychiatrist Michael McGrath has astutely noted, there has been virtually no scientific exploration of either codependency or dependent personality disorder [5].

A combination not only of life circumstances and interpersonal difficulties, but also of specific personality traits influenced by genetic and neurophysiological factors may predispose certain individuals to pathological altruism. Support for this is provided by Williams syndrome, a genetic disorder characterized by a sweetly trusting gullibility [7]. Differences in receptors related to oxytocin and vasopressin have been related to differing degrees of human trust and ruthlessness [8]. Hyperempathetic traits involving exceptionally sensitive abilities to feel the pain of others may also play a role in the "burn out" some people feel due to empathetic distress [9]. Such traits may also be affiliated with the increased rates of victimization seen in those who are excessively giving [10]. As Satoshi Kanazawa notes [11], selfless behavior underlies acceptance of abuse from a spouse in some situations, or acceptance of abuse from the self in others.

Altruism, particularly in its more perverted forms, can sometimes be found with a pernicious self-righteousness [12]. Self-righteous, or *apparent* altruism, can be seen in a wide variety of scenarios, ranging from political extremism to cancer caregiving. Those whose care for cancer patients reaches self-harming extremes turn out, interestingly, to be unable to comfortably receive care themselves [13].

Perhaps the most important personality traits underlying both healthy and pathological altruism are empathy and compassion. According to Klimecki and Singer [9], these are distinct concepts. Empathy involves experiencing the same feelings as the person with whom we are empathizing, somewhat like feeling bad for someone in a pit and climbing down into the pit to comfort. Compassion involves concern, but not necessarily the same feelings as the person to whom we are offering compassion, like inviting the person in a pit up to your level to share a cup of tea and talk more dispassionately about the problem together. Compassion, therefore, tends to foster adaptive forms of altruism, and empathy more pathological expressions of it [9]. It appears that people can learn to react in a compassionate rather than empathetic manner [14].

The fatigued nurse who leaves the profession because she empathizes too deeply with her suffering patients might be said to display pathological altruism. The same could be said of the selfless, sweet-natured daughter who devotes herself completely to her demanding mother's care, ultimately dying lonely, unappreciated, and without much-longed-for children of her own. All in all, pathological altruism can involve "an excessive expression of empathy demonstrated in ways that can interfere with rational social behaviors" [4].

Eating Disordered Individuals as Prototypical Pathological Altruists: Theory and Descriptions

"I was a pleaser from a very young age to my father, mother and other family members and friends, and this took away my freedom to make choices that were right for me," writes a 44-year-old woman in recovery from anorexia nervosa after over 20 years of illness (D. Friedman, personal communication, September 7, 2009). "I was the super woman at our local swim club where my kids swam. I did everything from ordering suits to running meets. I volunteered for every job, every week… The happiness of others was primary in my life."

There could hardly be a clearer example of pathological altruism. Individuals with eating disorders tend to be supreme givers. While in no way limited to people who go on to develop eating disorders, altruism seems to characterize this population. Often, a poorly defined sense of self leads those who develop eating disorders to constantly adapt themselves to external needs and expectations [15]. The experience of negating themselves and denying their needs in order to serve others therefore becomes all too familiar. Sufferers, therapists [16], researchers [17] and theoreticians [15] have all documented the low priority eating disorders patients allocate to their own rights and wishes and the high priority they give to the needs and expectations of others. People with anorexia nervosa think so much of other people and so little of themselves that others are often forced to take over the function of self-care.

The etiology of eating disorders is complex and multifactorial. Genetic, biological, temperamental, developmental, family, personality, sociocultural, interpersonal and circumstantial factors contribute collectively to risk. We should keep in mind that pathological altruism fits into a large puzzle and that its place in the full etiological picture is still poorly understood.

Gender is the most significant risk factor for an eating disorder, and the role of genetics is paramount [18]. Genes also play a role in altruism, which may share certain genetic pathways with eating disorders. A significant proportion of the differences between people's prosocial attitudes is due to heredity [19], and specific genes associated with altruism as measured by the Selflessness Scale (DRD4, IGF2 and DRD5) have been preliminarily identified [20]. What exactly may be passed on genetically is not clear. An inherited sensitivity factor associated with high empathy levels [9] may predispose some children to be more attuned to interpersonal cues and to take on responsibility for other's wellbeing. Inborn sensitivity may interact with other genetic and environmental factors to create vulnerability for an eating disorder.

Subjective and objective realities do not always correspond. Parents are not to be blamed for their children's eating disorder. The subjective experience of unmet needs may result from or be exaggerated by an extreme sensitivity to the social environment that has a primarily genetic, temperamental and/or biological base. Strober's conceptualization of anorexia nervosa, for example, involves a genetically-based personality style that inhibits natural exploration and easily leads to a mismatch between child and parenting style [21].

Hilde Bruch was among the first clinicians to emphasize the extent to which individuals with eating disorders, whom she called "consummate caretakers", stunt the growth of self-identity by constantly giving to others [22]. Clinicians and theorists from the self-psychology school have extended her views and placed particular emphasis on eating disordered patients as selfless souls serving others' needs. Heinz Kohut's self-psychology [23], in particular, provides us with a theory of development of pathological altruism as seen in the eating disorders.

To develop healthily, said Kohut, small children need to feel special and appreciated, or "mirrored" in the eyes of significant others. When told they are gorgeous and their scribbles masterpieces, when shown their opinions are valued and their needs legitimate, an "archaic grandiosity" that forms the basis of a cohesive sense of self and healthy self-esteem develops [23]. According to Kohut, when needs such as that for mirroring are not subjectively met early in life, children fail to develop the ability to turn to others in a healthy way and use them as "selfobjects", or people who serve the function of fulfilling others' needs [24]. An exaggerated need for responsiveness from others develops, and a sense of self-esteem that failed to crystallize during early childhood becomes less and less likely to be established. Compliments, acts of caring, and admiration for genuine virtues, intelligence, talents, skills or competencies often come to fall like water from a duck's back, leaving the youngster tragically starved for the very reinforcement being offered.

Sensitive children often cope with unmet needs they experience for care, holding, and understanding by severing and ignore them. They come to regard them as excessive and unjustified. They grow ashamed of their desire to be seen and acknowledged, ashamed of depending on others. Children who perceive their caretakers as burdened may strive very early on to lighten that burden by being undemanding and coping on their own. In extreme cases, it becomes top priority not to be a burden on anybody and a brittle façade of self-sufficiency sets in.

Eating disorders may be seen in this context as an attempt to deny dependence on everybody and everything, symbolized by them becoming dependent on food-related contexts. Other biological needs, such as the need for rest, sleep, and sex are often also pushed aside. Medical care may be seen as superfluous and basic interpersonal needs for affection, support and help are denied. A regimented, ritualized daily schedule regulated by behavioral and moral rules provides an effective strategy to avoid the satisfaction of genuine needs and to appear self-sufficient. Helping others often features high up on a long list of obligations.

Attempts to help others by lightening their burden begin at home. Bruch wrote that her patients with anorexia nervosa had spent their lives learning how to adapt themselves to others in order to lessen demands on them [22]. Palazzoli emphasized the guilt experienced by children who later develop eating disorders in response to their needs, and described family dynamics that lead them to feel responsible for their parents' wellbeing [25]. Bachar [26] pointed out that eating disordered patients often recall feeling responsible for their parents and taking on a comforting, organizing role at home.

The Pathological Nature of Altruism in Eating Disordered Individuals

Pathology in the Guise of Health

It is common in children and adolescents who go on to develop eating disorders for pathology to masquerade as health when it comes to altruism. Autonomy and self-sufficiency are all too often misinterpreted as signs of health and good adjustment by parents, peers, loved ones, colleagues, teachers and society at large. All too often the parents of adolescents with eating disorders, particularly anorexia nervosa, ignore and deny their child's illness as long as possible, and react with incredulity and disbelief when confronted with it. How, they ask, could such an easy, sweet-natured, undemanding and self-disciplined person possibly become ill?

Since contemporary society overvalues independence [27], autonomy can appear deceptively adaptive. A person who seems to be coping without help tends to be admired at the personal, familial, and broader cultural level. Pathological altruism, too, can look misleadingly healthy. Altruism is socially approved; parents, teachers, religious leaders, and society at large teach us the value of giving to family members, siblings, classmates, friends, and the needy. In narrative research, women with anorexia nervosa have talked about the encouragement they received from their families and their social and cultural environments to substitute others' needs for their own [17].

Why 'Pathological'?

So let us take a look at what renders the altruism that so often accompanies eating disorders pathological. A person with an eating disorder equates food with self-indulgence and selfishness. Eating healthily means caring for oneself, giving oneself sustenance, responding to inner needs and allowing oneself spontaneous pleasure, and all these things become problematic. In the absence of the ability to give to self and little sense of how much of self is reasonable to relinquish for the sake of others, giving often smacks of martyrdom.

The motivations and feelings behind the act of giving are central to the distinction between normal and pathological altruism. For people with eating disorders, the simple joy of giving is often tainted by anger and frustration, conscious or unconscious, at sacrificing so much and receiving so little in return. Bruch wrote that women with anorexia nervosa help and serve other people, but disown their anger and aggression [28]. The tendency of women with anorexia nervosa to repress needs and feelings, especially anger, to protect interpersonal relationships, has been supported from a cognitive and sociological perspective by Geller and her colleagues [29].

Inner values, experiences, initiatives and needs are often dismissed because of a need for acceptance and admiration [15]. Hilde Bruch pointed out that individuals with eating disorders often crave connections and wish to maintain them at all costs. They see giving to others and adjusting themselves to their expectations as a precondition for positive regard, acceptance, affection or love. They also fear feeling rejected and lost should a relationship be disrupted [22].

Despite the emotional price paid for constant compromise, however, pathological altruism has significant adaptive value for eating disorders patients, since in the short term its rewards mask and provide relief from feelings of worthlessness and inefficacy.

Research Supporting Pathological Altruism in Eating Disordered Individuals

Selflessness A self-report "Selflessness Scale" was developed by Bachar and his colleagues for use in empirical research, to measure the degree to which people forgo their own needs and serve the interests and well-being of others [30]. Research using this scale has shown that Selflessness Scores indeed distinguish between women with eating disorders and control women [30], are positively associated with the severity of anorexic symptomatology [31], and predict the development of eating pathology in adolescent schoolgirls with 82 % sensitivity and 63 % specificity.

Concern for Appropriateness This construct, measured by the self-report "Concern for Appropriateness Scale" [32], was conceived and first applied in the field of social psychology. It captures a social style involving constant efforts to read others' needs and expectations with the aim of evaluating and adopting appropriate behavioral strategies that will prevent the impression of standing out or appearing different from others. Concern for appropriateness has been found to be associated with a general tendency to notice and be influenced behaviorally by interpersonal and media messages [33].

In a study by the first author in which a large group of women with a present or past history of anorexia nervosa completed the Concern for Appropriateness Scale and a measure of sociocultural attitudes towards appearance, the women with a past or present eating disorder were more concerned with appropriateness than control women. Concern for Appropriateness Scores were positively associated with symptom severity [34].

External social circumstances therefore seem to take precedence over an internal compass of what is beneficial for the self in women with eating disorders. These results support Bruch's [28] observation that women with anorexia nervosa depend on external sources for their self-esteem and may become experts at reading cues from others about how to feel and behave. Vitousek and Ewald [35] emphasized the combined contribution of genetic and environmental factors to the failure to develop a clear sense of self, potentially leading to an over-reliance on social and environmental cues.

Desirable, socially "appropriate" values and behaviors vary sharply in different cultural settings and different historical periods. In contemporary Western societies, an ongoing strict diet of unrealistically thin women fed to us constantly via the media motivates many women to overvalue thinness and strive for it at all costs. In the study on Concern for Appropriateness mentioned above [34], it was therefore hypothesized that one of the social messages women highly concerned with social appropriateness tend to endorse is the importance of external appearance, and in particular of a thin body. Results supported this hypothesis: The association between concern for appropriateness and eating disorder symptomatology was fully mediated, or explained, by sociocultural attitudes towards appearance.

Cultural norms on physical appearance and the culturally "appropriate" body shape therefore seem to have far more influence on some women than others. Certain women particularly concerned with appropriateness may be motivated to attain a thin body shape even if they have to sacrifice their health to do so. Disturbed eating attitudes and behaviors, and in extreme cases an eating disorder, may develop as a consequence.

The cultural ideal of thinness takes on particular personal relevance during puberty. Adolescence is typically characterized by a preoccupation with appearance and identity development, heightening susceptibility to pressures and influences from the media [36]. Teenagers are heavy users of many forms of mass media, particularly magazines. It therefore hardly seems surprising that adolescence is the peak onset period for eating disorders.

Yet media influences are only one avenue for the transmission of sociocultural messages. Teenagers tend to be sensitive about appearance-related comments, and peer pressure peaks during adolescence. The vast majority of adolescent girls engage in dieting behavior in some form and being thin is part of today's aesthetic ideal. Girls who sacrifice their health to present a proscribed, desired body shape are paying a high price to fulfill a group requirement, give the group what it needs, seek approval and avoid being discounted. Conforming to a socio-cultural group ideal of thinness to the extent that an eating disorder develops can in itself be regarded as an expression of pathological altruism.

Concern for appropriateness is no doubt both environmentally and genetically based. It has been found to be associated with a vasopressin receptor AVPR1A promoter region microsatellite [37], and the same microsatellite was found to be associated with disordered eating [38]. Assuming a link between concern for appropriateness and pathological altruism, the vasopressin receptor gene may be contributing risk for anorexia, at least in part, via pathological altruism. This line of investigation should be further explored in future research.

The Anomaly Between Pathological Altruism and Narcissism

Freud defined altruism as "the opposite of egoism" [39], and indeed, the term is commonly used as an antonym of selfishness or narcissism. Yet despite eating disordered individuals' frequent surrender to others, they often describe themselves as narcissistic and selfish. Core symptoms of eating disorders such as self-destructive starvation, binge-eating, purging, defiant self-sufficiency, non-communication and social isolation appear manipulative, controlling and self-centered—so far removed from altruism, in fact, that they invariably trigger hostile reactions and earn eating disorder patients a reputation of being notoriously difficult to understand and treat [40]. Eating disordered patients are characterized not only by selflessness, but, paradoxically, by narcissism as well [41]. Rather than parading their virtues in a grandiose and forthright fashion, eating disordered patients tend to fit Gabbard's [42] description of "hypervigilant narcissists": "At the core of their inner world is a deep sense of shame related to their secret wish to exhibit themselves in a grandiose manner… Attention is continually directed toward others… they study others intensely to figure out how to behave." So if pathological altruism is a characteristic of eating disorders that needs to be addressed in treatment and recovery, how can it be reconciled with narcissism?

Narcissism and altruism may in fact represent two sides of the same coin. With the onset of an eating disorder, frustration at constantly giving so much, sacrificing so much of self, comes to a peak. One thing that can be held on to as one's own is food intake and a low weight. An eating disorder expresses the wish to be the center at least of a narrowly defined world. Symptoms of weight loss, remaining thin despite overeating, overcoming appetite, maintaining a dangerously low weight and/or purging without becoming ill [41] create the grandiose illusion of being empowered, special and superior to others. When they first start to lose weight, women with anorexia nervosa report feeling "delighted, inspired, triumphant, proud and powerful … special, superior and deserving of the respect and admiration of others" [43]. This initial "high" could conceivably be connected with changes in endorphin levels, associated with a feeling of elevation in athletes, and with changes in dopamine levels, associated with increased reward [44, 45].

Food consumption is viewed as selfish by those with eating disorders, and self-starvation is experienced as depriving, selfless, and therefore, paradoxically, nourishing and satisfying. Fasting has historically been a means of drawing close to the Divine in most religions. In eating disorders, as in extreme forms of religion, self-indulgence and pleasures of the flesh tend to be shunned [46]. Freedom from body and bodily needs can lead to a feeling of immortality, omnipotence, spiritual purity and moral superiority. A sense of satisfaction and triumph is achieved by relinquishing parts of oneself [47]. Autonomy and self-sufficiency are valued (after thinness) above all else, and despite its toll, giving to others becomes one of the only permissible sources of pleasure.

Implications for Recovery, Treatment and Prevention

The pathological altruism associated with eating disorder symptomatology has important implications for recovery, treatment and prevention. Treatment is an unfamiliar and challenging experience for eating disorder patients, since it provides the opportunity to focus on their needs instead of those of others. One potential trap for therapists lies in the character of pathological altruism itself; patients may be hypersensitive to the therapists' reactions, suggestions, expectations and narcissistic needs, tending to respond "appropriately" instead of exploring and expressing genuine feelings and problems. Objectives of therapy extend well beyond the achievement of a healthy weight, body image and eating habits. Therapeutic goals should include learning to recognize and fulfill authentic needs, developing and consolidating a stable and coherent sense of identity, learning to distinguish and respect clear boundaries between self and other, finding the courage to differ, and acquiring the ability to buffer vulnerability and to counteract negative messages from the media, teachers, friends and family.

During genuine recovery from an eating disorder, with or without the help of therapy, pathological aspects of altruism are usually shed, and the act of giving no longer diminishes or ignores integrity, beliefs, values needs or a sense of genuineness. Cross-sectional research has shown the levels of selflessness and concern for appropriateness in women completely recovered from anorexia nervosa to be similar to those of women with no history of an eating disorder [31, 34]. Pathological altruism therefore may be an aspect of an eating disorder that can, thankfully, gradually heal with recovery from eating and weight symptoms as the individual develops a sense of self and the ability to place appropriate boundaries between self and others.

The overlap between pathological altruism and eating disorders has also potential implications in the field of prevention. Further research should examine and clarify whether, and how specifically, pathological altruism predicts the emergence of an eating disorder as opposed to other psychopathology such as depression, anxiety or obsessive-compulsive disorder. In the meantime, much anecdotal, clinical, narrative and empirical evidence suggests that pathological altruism may be a precursor of, and therefore a risk factor, for eating disorders. Parents, teachers, coaches, doctors, and the public at large should be educated and trained to be on the lookout for overly giving, self-sacrificing children and teenagers. The aim of such training would be to increase awareness that such individuals may be experiencing serious and undetected distress. Pathological altruism, if detected early enough, may play a role in providing a valuable warning about the threat of an impending eating disorder. Such a warning sign, together with other risk factors such as specific personality traits and genetic markers yet to be identified in prospective research, could be incorporated into a recognized risk profile for eating disorders. If high risk can be detected, preemptive interventions such as individual psychotherapy, family therapy, nutritional counseling, psychoeducation, assertiveness training, changes in the social or study environment, and acts on behalf of the society at large to reduce the amount of thin-ideal advertisements in the media, may all be able to prevent the enormous pain and suffering inflicted by an eating disorder, and possibly even save lives.

Take Home Points

- Individuals with eating disorders tend to sacrifice their own needs and interests and devote themselves instead to helping and serving others.
- The major motivations for giving in healthy altruism are openness to new experiences and a desire for personal growth. In contrast, the major motivation for giving in eating-disordered individuals is to please others, gain approval, and avoid criticism and rejection.

- Pathologically altruistic behavior that stems from a lack of a sense of self involves reading, anticipating, or guessing others' needs and giving them priority over one's own.
- People concerned with appropriateness may be more vigilant than others concerning cultural norms on physical appearance and the culturally "appropriate" body shape, motivating them to attain it at any price, even if they have to sacrifice their health to do so.
- The autonomy and altruism of children and adolescents who go on to develop eating disorders are all too often misinterpreted as signs of health and good adjustment by parents, peers, other loved ones, colleagues, teachers, and society at large.
- Women with anorexia nervosa often feel they were encouraged by their families and cultural environments to substitute others' needs for their own.
- Much anecdotal, clinical, narrative, and empirical evidence suggests that pathological altruism may be a precursor of, and therefore a risk factor, for eating disorders.
- Pathological altruism may be an aspect of an eating disorder that, thankfully, can heal with recovery from eating and weight symptoms.

References

1. Moll J, Schulkin J. Social attachment and aversion in human moral cognition. Neurosci Biobehav Rev. 2009;33:456–65.
2. Seelig BJ, Rosof L. Normal and pathological altruism. J Am Psychoanal Assoc. 2001;49:933–59.
3. Oakley B, Knafo A, Madhavan G, Wilson DS, editors. Pathological altruism. New York: Oxford University Press; 2012.
4. Perlin M. Considering pathological altruism in the law from therapeutic jurisprudence and neuroscience perspectives. In: Oakley B, Knafo A, Madhavan G, Wilson DS, editors. Pathological altruism. New York: Oxford University Press; 2012.
5. McGrath M. Codependency and Pathological Altruism. In: Oakley B, Knafo A, Madhavan G, Wilson DS, editors. Pathological altruism. New York: Oxford University Press; 2012.
6. Stone MH. Normal narcissism: an etiological and ethological perspective. In: Ronningstam CF, editor. Disorders of narcissism. Northvale (NJ): Jason Aronson; 2000. p. 7–28.
7. Riby DM, Bruce V, Jawaid A. Everyone's friend? The case of Williams syndrome. In: Oakley B, Knafo A, Madhavan G, Wilson DS, editors. Pathological altruism. New York: Oxford University Press; 2012.
8. Knafo A, Israel S, Darvasi A, Bachner-Melman R, Uzefovsky F, Cohen L, et al. Individual differences in allocation of funds in the dictator game associated with length of the arginine vasopressin 1a receptor RS3 promoter region and correlation between RS3 length and hippocampal mRNA. Genes Brain Behav. 2008;7:266–75.
9. Klimecki O, Singer T. Empathic distress fatigue rather than compassion fatigue?—Integrating findings from empathy research in psychology and social neuroscience. In: Oakley B, Knafo A, Madhavan G, Wilson DS, editors. Pathological altruism. New York: Oxford University Press; 2012.

10. Homant R, Kennedy D. Does no good deed go unpunished? The victimology of altruism. In: Oakley B, Knafo A, Madhavan G, Wilson DS, editors. Pathological altruism. New York: Oxford University Press; 2012.
11. Kanazawa S. Battered women, happy genes: there is no such thing as altruism, pathological or otherwise. In: Oakley B, Knafo A, Madhavan G, Wilson DS, editors. Pathological altruism. New York: Oxford University Press; 2012.
12. Brin D. Self-addiction and self-righteousness. In: Oakley B, Knafo A, Madhavan G, Wilson DS, editors. Pathological altruism. New York: Oxford University Press; 2012.
13. Li M, Rodin G. Altruism and suffering in the context of cancer caregiving: implications of a relational paradigm. In: Oakley B, Knafo A, Madhavan G, Wilson DS, editors. Pathological altruism. New York: Oxford University Press; 2012.
14. Decety J, Michalska KJ. Neural circuits subserving empathy and sympathy in typically developing children and children with social behavior disorders. In: Oakley B, Knafo A, Madhavan G, Wilson DS, editors. Pathological altruism. New York: Oxford University Press; 2012.
15. Goodsitt A. Eating disorders: a self psychological perspective. In: Garner DM, Garfinkel PE, editors. Handbook of psychotherapy for eating disorders. New York: Guilford Press; 1997. p. 205–28.
16. Minuchin S, Rosman BL, Baker L. Psychosomatic families: anorexia nervosa in context. Cambridge (MA): Harvard University Press; 1987.
17. Wechselblatt T, Gurnick G, Simon R. Autonomy and relatedness in the development of anorexia nervosa: a clinical case series using grounded theory. Bull Menninger Clin. 2000;64:91–123.
18. Klump K, Kaye W, Strober M. The evolving genetic foundations of eating disorders. Psychiatr Clin North Am. 2001;24:215–25.
19. Asbury K, Dunn J, Pike A, Plomin R. Nonshared environmental influences on individual differences in early behavioral development: a monozygotic twin differences study. Child Dev. 2003;74:933–43.
20. Bachner-Melman R, Gritsenko I, Nemanov L, Zohar AH, Dina C, Ebstein RP. Dopaminergic polymorphisms associated with self-report measures of human altruism: a fresh phenotype for the dopamine D4 receptor. Mol Psy. 2005;10:333–5.
21. Strober M. Disorders of the self in anorexia nervosa: an organismic-developmental paradigm. In: Johnson C, editor. Psychodynamic treatment of anorexia nervosa and bulimia. New York: Guilford Press; 1991. p. 354–73.
22. Bruch H. The golden cage: the enigma of anorexia nervosa. Cambridge (MA): Harvard University Press; 1978.
23. Kohut H. The analysis of the self. New York: International Universities Press; 1971.
24. Kohut H. The psychoanalytic treatment of narcissistic personality disorders. Psychoanal Study Child. 1968;23:86–113.
25. Selvini Palazzoli M. Self Starvation. New York: Jason Aronson; 1978.
26. Bachar E. The contributions of self psychology to the treatment of anorexia and bulimia. Am J Psychother. 1998;52:147–65.
27. Fineman MA. The autonomy myth: a theory of dependency. New York: New Press; 2005.
28. Bruch H. Eating disorders: Obesity, anorexia nervosa and the person within. London: Routledge and Kegan Paul; 1973.
29. Geller J, Cockell SJ, Goldner EM, Flett GL. Inhibited expression of negative emotions and interpersonal orientation in anorexia nervosa. Int J Eat Disord. 2000;28:8–19.
30. Bachar E, Canetti L, Latzer Y, Gur E, Berry E, Bonne O. Rejection of life in anorexic and bulimic patients. Int J Eat Disord. 2002;31:42–7.
31. Bachner-Melman R, Zohar AH, Ebstein RP, Bachar E. The relationship between selflessness levels and the severity of anorexia nervosa symptomatology. Eur Eat Disord Rev. 2007;15:213–20.
32. Lennox RD, Wolfe RN. Revision of the Self-Monitoring Scale. J Pers Soc Psychol. 1984;46:1349–64.

33. Johnson MA. Concern for appropriateness scale and behavioral conformity. J Pers Assess. 1989;53:567–74.
34. Bachner-Melman R, Zohar AH, Elizur Y, Kremer I, Golan M, Ebstein RP. Protective self-presentation style: association with disordered eating and anorexia nervosa mediated by sociocultural attitudes to appearance. Eat Weight Disord. 2009;14:1–12.
35. Vitousek K, Ewald L. Self-representation in eating disorders: a cognitive perspective. In: Segal Z, Blatt S, editors. The self in emotional disorders. New York: Guildford Press; 1993. p. 221–57.
36. Wertheim EH, Paxton SJ, Schultz HK, Muir SL. Why do adolescent girls watch their weight? An interview study examining sociocultural pressures to be thin. J Psychol Res. 1997;42:345–55.
37. Bachner-Melman R, Zohar AH, Bacon-Shnoor N, Elizur Y, Nemanov L, Gritsenko I, et al. Linkage between vasopressin receptor AVPRIA promoter region microsatellites and measures of social behavior in man. J Individ Dif. 2005;26:2–10.
38. Bachner-Melman R, Zohar AH, Elizur Y, Nemanov L, Gritsenko I, Konis D, et al. Association between a vasopressin receptor AVPRIA promoter region microsatellite and eating behavior measured by a self-report questionnaire (eating attitudes test) in a family-based study of a non-clinical population. Int J Eat Disord. 2004;36:451–60.
39. Freud S. Introductory lectures on psychoanalysis: the libido theory and narcissism. In: Strachey J, editor and translator. The standard edition of the complete psychological works of Sigmund Freud. London: Hogarth Press; 1957 (Original work published 1917). Vol. 16, p. 412–30.
40. Kaplan AS, Garfinkel PE. Difficulties in treating patients with eating disorders: a review of patient and clinician variables. Can J Psychiatry. 1999;44:665–70.
41. Riebel L. Hidden grandiosity in bulimics. Theor Res Pract Train. 2000;37:180–8.
42. Gabbard GO. Two subtypes of narcissistic personality disorder. Bull Menninger Clin. 1989;53:527–32.
43. Bemis K. A comparison of the subjective experience of individuals with eating disorders and phobic disorders [dissertation]. Minnesota (MN): Univ. of Minnesota; 1986.
44. Bachner-Melman R, Lerer E, Zohar AH, Kremer I, Elizur Y, Nemanov L, et al. Anorexia nervosa, perfectionism and dopamine D4 receptor (DRD4). Am J Med Genet B Neuropsychiatr Genet. 2007;144:748–56.
45. Barry VC, Klawans HL. On the role of dopamine in the pathophysiology of anorexia nervosa. J Neural Transm. 1976;38:107–22.
46. Lelwica M. The religion of thinness: satisfying the spiritual hungers behind women's obsession with food and weight. Carlsbad (CA): Gürze Books; 2009.
47. Green A. Life narcissism death narcissism. London: Free Association Books; 2001.

Chapter 8
Women with Eating Disorders and a History of Sexual Abuse: An Integrative Treatment Approach

Eynat Zubery, Yael Latzer and Daniel Stein

Abstract This chapter proposes a practice-based model for the treatment of patients with eating disorders (EDs) in the context of a history of childhood sexual abuse (CSA). Our integrated ED-CSA treatment model includes 3 phases. The first acute phase focuses on the stabilization of ED-related symptomatology and reduction of other health threatening behaviors. When this is achieved, patients move on to the second phase involving treatment of trauma-related issues. The third phase focuses on further integration of material previously elicited in the course of treatment. Treatment can be terminated if the patient is considered symptomatically stabilized and if trauma-related material has been worked through at least to some extent. Otherwise, a fourth intervention phase focusing on either general functioning or additional trauma-related work may be indicated. This model is fundamentally about the need to empower the patients. This is achieved by reducing their social isolation and sense of helplessness and expanding the range of adaptive options offered for effective coping with trauma-related issues. This model further assumes that ED symptoms have to be stabilized to some extent before trauma-related issues can be treated. It is considered that following these interventions, patients will no longer have to rely on ED-related and other health-endangering behaviors for trauma-related affect regulation. The important contribution of this model is its

E. Zubery (✉)
Head of Eating Disorders treatment and Research Center, Hanotrim,
Shalvata Mental Health Center, Raanana, Israel
e-mail: eynat@dr-zubery.co.il

E. Zubery · D. Stein
The Sackler Faculty of Medicine, Tel Aviv University, Tel Aviv, Israel

Y. Latzer
Faculty of Social Welfare and Health Sciences, Haifa University, Haifa, Israel

Y. Latzer
Director of Eating Disorder Institute, Rambam Healthcare Campus, Haifa, Israel

D. Stein
Pediatric Psychosomatic Department Safra Children's Hospital, Chaim Sheba Medical
Center, Tel Hashomer, Ramat Gan, Israel

Y. Latzer and D. Stein (eds.), *Bio-Psycho-Social Contributions to Understanding Eating Disorders*, DOI 10.1007/978-3-319-32742-6_8

applicability for the treatment of ED patients both with and without a history of CSA. Further research is needed to establish the utility and implications of this treatment in the overall management of combined ED and CSA.

Introduction

Clinicians in the field of eating disorders (EDs), particularly feminist-oriented therapists, have argued for years that child sexual abuse (CSA) is a significant risk factor for the development of an ED [1–4]. It had been further noted that symptoms exhibited by women with history of sexual abuse may markedly overlap with those exhibited by women with an ED, likely including preoccupations with body shape, food and weight, and behaviors such as self-starvation and binge/purge (B/P) cycles. They are conceptualized to serve as a form of dissociation to facilitate psychic numbing and avoidance of trauma-related contents and behaviors, and to decrease trauma-associated hyper-arousal [1–4].

Over the past two decades, researchers have established that CSA may be a significant, albeit nonspecific risk factor for the development and maintenance of an ED [5–13]. Lifetime prevalence rates of patients who present with both an ED and a history of sexual/physical abuse may vary from 18–85 %, reflecting considerable discrepancies in the definitions of traumatic/abusive experiences and the considerable difficulty in supporting the validity of abuse reports [3, 7, 9, 13–15].

Patients with EDs and a history of CSA commonly exhibit diverse psychiatric comorbidities, in particular mood, anxiety, somatoform and dissociative disorders. In addition, disorders related to impulse dyscontrol, including self-inflicted injuries, suicidal tendencies, risk-taking behaviors and addictions are highly common in people with comorbid ED and abuse history. Consequently, the prognosis of these individuals tends to be less favorable; moreover, a history of abuse has been associated with treatment failure where issues related to the abuse remain unaddressed [9].

The aim of the present chapter is to propose a practice-based intervention model integrating knowledge accumulated by ED and CSA experts. Firstly, we present an updated review of the literature on the relationship between ED and CSA. This will be followed by a review of treatment models for ED patients with a history of CSA. Lastly, we describe our proposed practice-based model for the treatment of combined ED-CSA pathology.

The Relationship Between EDs and CSA

A key finding in the study of the relationship between EDs and CSA is related to the postulated role of abuse events in the predisposition to and maintenance of an ED. Thus, abuse events may occur several years before the clinical presentation of the ED [12]. Secondly, the overall prognosis of an ED is less favorable when associated with a history of CSA [16].

Thirdly, a history of CSA is associated more frequently with binge/purge (B/P)-type EDs, including anorexia nervosa, B/P–type (AN-B/P), bulimia nervosa (BN), and eating disorders not otherwise specified (EDNOS) with B/P behaviors, than with restricting-type AN (AN-R) or EDNOS [6–8, 13, 17, 18]. The latter group may report a history of sexual and/or physical traumatization as often as healthy controls [19]. These findings are supported by prospective longitudinal studies showing that CSA in an important predictor of B/P symptoms [20], and by large-scale meta-analyses (combining 53 studies altogether) supporting the associations between CSA and B/P type EDs [12, 21]. Still other studies have not found a higher incidence of CSA in patients with BN [22]. One possible explanation for this discrepancy is that the effects of childhood traumatization may interact with personality characteristics associated with the AN-BP subtype rather than with characteristics associated with the AN-R subtype, particularly the tendency to exhibit greater mood lability and impulsive behaviors [19]. Lastly, a history of traumatic experiences has been associated with the development of multiple comorbid conditions in patients with EDs in addition to the ED per se [6, 8, 9, 23, 24].

Note that trauma history in patients with EDs is usually substantiated only after an extended period of treatment [4, 7, 15, 25], at a point when ED- and trauma-related symptoms regularly interact with and influence each other [22]. Similarly, the unusually high rates of sexual assault during late adolescence or early adulthood in women with BN [1, 26] may suggest that this later abuse may represent a marker of earlier, as yet repressed or undisclosed, CSA [27].

Similarities in the Symptomatology of EDs and CSA

Patients with EDs and CSA victims share many clinical and psychological features. Sexual abuse may cause and intensify body hatred, body shame and body image distortion, all highly characteristic also of ED-related pathology. Moreover, similar to CSA victims, patients with EDs tend to refer to their body as a "battleground" [3]. Both groups may attempt to subdue sexual impulses, avoid interpersonal relationships, and obtain "safe" caretaking, while simultaneously "forget" the existence of their body and inflict self-punishment when feeling overwhelmed [25]. Poor recognition of hunger and satiety may appear as a result of psychic numbing aimed to counteract hyper-arousal or avoid painful emotions. Furthermore, the attitude of CSA victims toward food and eating resembles that of patients with EDs: both describe their food rituals as a "shameful secret" and exhibit fear of discovery that may resemble their attitudes toward sexuality, often leading to considerable isolation. Finally, the use of B/P behaviors to temporarily reduce mental pain in patients with EDs, whether with a history of CSA or not, may be in many ways similar to the function of self-mutilation and abuse behaviors [28] in both conditions.

In addition, both patients with EDs and victims of CSA may share deep-seated constellations of interpersonal difficulties, including deprived, diffuse, or unstable identity, interpersonal ineffectiveness and a sense of powerlessness, mistrust or insecurity in relationships. Both groups also reveal a limited sense of safety and security, and exhibit fear of abandonment, intrusion and intimacy, and confusion regarding their internal and interpersonal boundaries [22]. Other shared symptoms include deficits in impulse and affect regulation and in self-soothing, alexithymia, and concrete communication patterns [25].

Dissociation is particularly common in the presentation of victims of CSA. Operating as a defense mechanism, it is manifested via a variety of symptoms, including de-realization, de-personalization, ignoring pain, auditory hallucinations, and memory loss [29]. Dissociation may help traumatized individuals to cope with unbearable psychological distress, as it reduces awareness of trauma-related intrusive thoughts, memories, feelings, actions, and unaccepted sense of self [30, 31].

Many patients with EDs, mostly those diagnosed with B/P behaviors, have dissociative symptoms, particularly in the context of a history of sexual abuse, and/or comorbid borderline psychopathology. The dissociative symptoms manifested by patients with EDs likely include dissociation of feelings, body, thoughts, memories, and sensations, de-personalization and de-realization, as well as temporal distortion and instability, affective incongruity and instability, and addictive behaviors such as substance abuse and self-injurious behaviors (SIBs) [15, 31].

Finally, health-related and psychosomatic complaints are over-reported by both women with a history of sexual abuse and women with an ED. These include gastrointestinal complaints, abdominal pain, headache, other neurological symptoms, and muscle pain, as well as genital complaints, in particular difficulties in sexual functioning and pregnancy-related disturbances [32].

Integrative Treatment Strategies in Patients with an EDs and a History of CSA

The ED literature does not distinguish between different kinds of trauma; rather, it refers generally to "traumatized patients with EDs", "ED patients with comorbid PTSD", of "ED patients with past traumatic experiences" [9].

Although CSA is the most frequent cause of trauma among women diagnosed with an ED [33, 34], there is only a small body of literature suggesting specific ED-CSA integrative treatment models. Rather, current research emphasizes the integration of evidence-based effective treatments for PTSD and other trauma-related comorbidity into ED treatment programs, assuming that patients will be generally willing to begin trauma-related work once their ED-related symptoms and other maladaptive behaviors have subsided. Once nutritional rehabilitation occurs and some anxiety reduction skills are acquired, patients with EDs may be able to process emotional and cognitive trauma-related information [6, 8, 9]. By that time, they may be able to recover previously forgotten traumatic experiences, and previously dissociated abuse memories may emerge spontaneously. Moreover, once their cognitive setting is altered with the stabilization of weight and maladaptive consummatory behaviors, patients with EDs may perceive past experiences as abusive, leading to the emergence of inhibited PTSD symptoms [33].

Cognitive behavioral therapy (CBT) is the most empirically supported treatment for B/P type EDs, as well as for trauma-related comorbidities, including mood, anxiety, and substance use disorders. Prolonged exposure along with cognitive reprocessing and restructuring has been found beneficial for patients with PTSD [9, 35–37]. In more resistant cases, CBT can serve as the basis upon which other interventions, such as interpersonal psychotherapy, pharmacotherapy, family therapy, and psychodynamic therapy may be introduced [38–40]. From a different perspective, dialectical behavior therapy (DBT) has been used successfully in patients with EDs of the B/P type who are additionally diagnosed with borderline personality disorder and related conditions [41]. It may be of specific relevance for patients with coexisting B/P ED symptomatology and CSA who often present with disturbances responsive to DBT, including affective dysregulation [41], impulse control disorders, dissociative disorders [42], and PTSD [43–45]. Lastly, the Structural Process Model (SPM) based on the self-regulation theory may be effective in the treatment of complex, multi-symptomatic patients with ED and trauma history [25, 45–48]. In this model, the therapist acts as a mentor possessing expertise in recovery skills and strategies. Self-destructive symptoms are conceptualized as maladaptive self-regulatory behaviors that need be reduced by acquiring skills such as competency, control, hopefulness, choice and empowerment.

Persons [49], Zayfert and Becker [50] describe a case formulation approach that can be used to integrate empirically supported treatments for various co-existing conditions. In this approach, the clinician integrates hypotheses about the mechanisms causing and maintaining problematic behaviors that functionally link co-existing disorders with empirically validated therapeutic approaches for each disorder. Brewerton [9] argues that in this approach, empirical treatments such as CBT for EDs and PTSD can be integrated alongside a range of interventions that can be tailored for each disorder. This integrative approach is applied to patients with EDs in an attempt to deal with PTSD and other common trauma-related comorbid disorders.

When applying trauma-related integrative approaches in the management of EDs, the clinician should adhere to the treatment principles of both EDs and trauma. This is recommended because of the high prevalence of CSA in patients with ED and their overlapping symptoms. From a different perspective, when treating patients with CSA in general, including those with comorbid EDs, it is important to distinguish between an adult trauma which interferes with an already existing personality structure and childhood trauma, which shapes and distorts the developing personality. Integrative therapeutic approaches, although relevant for traumas at any age, are particularly suitable for complex PTSD (CPTSD) [51]—resulting from recurring or continuous trauma that usually starts at an early age. In CPTSD, the range of psychiatric disorders is considerably broader and more intricate in comparison with one-time PTSD conditions. Survivors of continuous trauma, especially if it starts at an early age, might develop a significant disturbance in personality constellation, including poor communication skills and severe identity disorders. These patients are at a high risk for re-victimization and recurring self- and other-inflicted injuries, and may present with severe disturbances in emotion regulation, self-awareness, and self-perception, including the lack of perception of themselves as victims. They may also suffer from maladaptive interpersonal relations and adverse alterations in their meaning systems [51, 52]. It comes as no surprise that such a prolonged and diffuse disturbance in almost every aspect of the trauma survivor's personality calls for complex integrative treatment interventions, such as those proposed in our model for comorbid CPTSD and EDs.

The Proposed Integrative Model: Background and Rationale

The idea underlying our integrative treatment approach is to routinely apply principles of CSA treatment to the treatment of EDs in general irrespective of whether they had, or had not experienced past CSA. In addition, it is important to distinguish between single trauma (PTSD) and recurring or continuous trauma such as CPTSD in the treatment of co-existing of EDs with PTSD. Surprisingly, only a relatively few studies have hitherto addressed the treatment of combined CPTSD-ED. Furthermore, to the best of our knowledge, there are no specific guidelines for the treatment of ED pathology in patients with comorbid CSA. Similarly, there are no specific guidelines for the pharmacological treatment of patients with combined ED-CPTSD [24].

Our integrated ED-CSA treatment model relies on theoretical and treatment recommendations of leading CSA experts, including Courtois [32, 34], Herman [51], Seligman [53], Gur [54] and Steele [55]. Herman [51] suggests that a core feature of the traumatic experience is a sense of disempowerment, detachment and isolation from significant others. Accordingly, the fundamentals of integrative CPTSD treatment lie in empowering the survivors and reversing their sense of lack of control, while establishing new relations with significant others [51]. Accordingly, any intervention by which power is again taken away from the traumatized patient by significant others, including therapists, may interfere with recovery.

According to Herman [51], therapists trained in the medical model may find it difficult to fully understand and accept the importance of personal empowerment in the therapeutic relationship with patients with CSA. This is particularly relevant in the medical and nutritional rehabilitation of patients with combined ED-CPTSD because the severity and immediacy of the physical and mental state may require therapists to intervene against the patients' will, in a manner potentially interfering with their sense of empowerment. Accordingly, treatment of an ED that does not take its potential effect on CPTSD into due account, could interfere, according to this line of thinking, with the therapeutic process, despite the obvious necessity in terms of physical health.

Patients with an ED and a history of CSA may exhibit a multitude of diverse and severe psychiatric comorbidities [9], may be misdiagnosed with borderline personality disorder, and may present with impairment in avoiding re-victimization. Moreover, they are often mistrustful and reluctant to receive treatment, and tend not to complete their treatment [6, 23], this likely interfering with the therapeutic process and leading to further deterioration. The need to formulate an integrative treatment model for patients with coexisting ED and a history of CSA is based not only on the resemblance of both disorders in terms of their psychiatric comorbidity and symptomatology, but also on the difficulty, in both conditions, in establishing adequate therapeutic relationships, further exacerbating the patients' sense of stigmatization and alienation [6, 9].

In order to offer a more effective therapeutic approach for combined ED-CPTSD along these lines, experts in the treatment of CSA were involved in the training of the multidisciplinary team of the Eating Disorders Outpatient Clinic at the Davidson Hanotrim Center in Raanana, Israel. During the training process, many therapists realized that about half of their patients actually had a history of CSA, and that in some cases it was the CSA that triggered the ED. The process involved joint reviews of the clinic's history of therapeutic failures as part of the training. The CSA experts emphasized that in many cases survivors of trauma fail to seek therapy not on account of the abuse per se, but rather due to resulting emotional, behavioral, or physical problems. Moreover, most patients would not talk about their CSA unless the therapist has made a clear reference to it and expressed a genuine wish to listen to the patient's story [1]. Finally, a great number of patients reported of sharing their CSA history only admitted to an inpatient or daycare program, where they might have felt safer.

Specific Therapeutic Considerations

Several issues to be considered in the treatment of patients with comorbid ED-CSA have arisen as a result of this training process, leading to revision of the treatment protocol:

1. Difficulty with maintaining the treatment regimen.
2. Treating SIBs, their dissociative functions, and issues of re-victimization—which are of particular importance in patients with comorbid ED-CSA, as these problems may be associated with a less favorable outcome.
3. Resistance to parental involvement by younger patients diagnosed with both an ED and CSA.
4. In the course of treatment, difficulties in reconstructing the trauma experience in the transference and countertransference processes.

1. Difficulty with maintaining the treatment regimen.

Therapists who treat patients with combined ED and CSA may experience repeated difficulties in maintaining the treatment framework and content. Throughout the treatment process, these patients may not to adhere to the treatment schedule and not to arrive on time to therapy sessions, as well as to cancel appointments at the last minute and then make urgent phone calls demanding to be seen immediately. Whereas these difficulties are typical for victims of CSA, the reluctance of patients with AN to engage in treatment and the symptomatic and behavioral instability of patients with BN, might exacerbate the lack of adherence to treatment even further. Moreover, there is an inherent difficulty in enhancing the compliance of patients with EDs with their nutritional and weight maintenance regimen. The maintenance of a well-defined setting in the treatment of ED patients with regard to place and time as well as to the ED-related regimen is clearly of considerable importance. Still, traumatized patients may require more flexibility and creativity in establishing the therapeutic setting with respect to both the conditions of treatment (e.g., allowing email correspondence), and to the ED-related regimen (e.g., considering the influence of flashbacks and dissociation on the patients' ability to adhere to their treatment plan).

2. Treatment of SIBs, their dissociative functions, and re-victimization.

When our ED treatment center was first opened in 1992, we insisted on a very explicit pre-treatment contract with the patients in which they undertook not to engage in self-harm behaviors. We further referred the patients to an emergency room whenever they engaged in SIBs in order to set firm boundaries and prevent these behaviors from recurring. Unfortunately, this approach failed in reducing the occurrence of SIBs. Furthermore, in many cases the patients were likely to expose their traumatic contents prematurely and unexpectedly during treatment or outside the therapy session, when their ED symptoms were still unstable, leading, in turn, to a host of acute regressive reactions, including SIBs.

Gradually, in an attempt to reduce these regressive phenomena, both the treatment team and the patients have reached the understanding that in the case of CSA, as part of the therapeutic process, dissociation can sometimes serve a temporary protective function in keeping painful traumatic experiences at bay. This understanding has led the patients to gradually share their daydreams and trance states, both during and outside the treatment sessions. Still, the understanding that the self-regulating potential of dissociation is reached at the expense of precipitating SIBs and other maladaptive behaviors has led to the introduction of DBT as part of the treatment protocol. The aim of DBT in this case has been to assist the traumatized patients in acquiring more adaptive means when affected by dysregulated thought patterns and emotions hitherto requiring immediate detachment.

3. Resistance to parental involvement by younger traumatized patients.

Our family-based treatment model focusing on parental involvement [56, 57] has proven effective in treating adolescents, and in some cases also young adults, with an ED. In keeping with the recommendations of the Maudsley Family-Based Treatment [FBT; 58, 59], parents have been required to supervise the patient's meals as an essential part of the treatment plan. We have found this parental involvement as highly beneficial in the management of the ED, failing to realize, at the time, that in some cases the parents might have actually been the abusers.

A case in point was a 25 year-old patient with severe AN-B/P type. At the time of her admission, she was a heavy laxative abuser (100 pills a day), exhibited recurrent SIBs, and was preoccupied with severe suicidal ideation. During her treatment she reported having experienced sexual abuse by one of her father's employees, and later by her brother. When no proof was found for her claims, she was thought to be experiencing false memories [60]. When her condition subsequently deteriorated to reach immediate risk of her health, the team considered involving her parents with supervision during and after her meals. The patient had mixed feelings about this plan. On one hand, she refused to call her father by name, to sit on chairs previously used by him at home, or to eat in his presence. On the other, she expressed a wish to spend quality time with him. This ambivalent behavior kept the team at bay for a time. We brought in external facilitators experienced in the treatment of CSA to review the case, and they recommended suspending all parental involvement. Shortly thereafter, the patient decided to stop her treatment in our center. A few months later, we received a call from a gynecologist to whom she had confided the occurrence of sexual abuse by her father. She agreed to return to our center for treatment, expressing extreme anger at the team for involving her parents in her treatment.

4. Difficulties in reconstructing the trauma experience in the transference and counter transference processes.

Therapists who treat patients with a history of abuse might inadvertently collude with the patients' avoidance of disclosing their abuse in an attempt to protect them. In essence, the patient might engage the therapist in the re-enactment of early parental inaction, in which the disclosed abuse might be repeatedly forgotten, ignored or minimized. Vicarious traumatization can become very real for therapists engaging in trauma-related work, and patient issues may often trigger therapists' concerns. Containment of both negative and positive transference and counter-transference processes thus seems vital for overcoming these patient-therapist obstacles [1]. The reluctance to disclose CSA-related history might be more powerful in patients with EDs, who might be reluctant to disclose both their ED-related symptoms and their abuse-related memories. As far as the therapists are concerned, this double "resistance" may render them even more cautious not to risk fragile therapeutic alliances with attempts to gather information, even if such information is vital for the treatment.

To resolve these dilemmas, a revised treatment protocol was gradually adopted in our center. Most importantly, the need to empower the patients, even those considered at risk as a result of their ED, was acknowledged. Patients were encouraged to actively participate in planning their treatment, including the proposed plan for meal supervision. The team took into account that some patients experiencing CSA would not disclose their abuse history until late in the treatment process, despite the potential for the reenactment of traumatic experiences during treatment.

Basic Treatment Structure and Principles of the Proposed Model

The Treatment Setting

Most of the referrals to our treatment center occur in the context of some resistance. The majority of the patients (around 70 %) enter the clinic accompanied by a significant other. We aim for the setting itself to provide a holding environment for the patient, her significant others, and the treatment providers. For this purpose, all team members (individual and family psychotherapists, dietitians, nurses and psychiatrists) work on the same days and hours, and patients are seen by the same multidisciplinary team from the start and at every visit. Transference and countertransference processes can thus be shared by different team members as well as by the entire team [56, 57].

Patient Evaluation

The patient is interviewed by a multidisciplinary team after filling out questionnaires designed to assess the type and severity of the ED, comorbid disorders, trauma and dissociation. The patient is interviewed separately without other family members being in the room. This gives the patient and her family an initial indication of our therapeutic rationale.

In the first session, a nurse evaluates the patient's medical and nutritional condition. The patient is asked about health-related issues and physical symptoms that may occur in the context of an ED and past abuse. These include gastrointestinal complaints, abdominal pain, headache, neurological problems, muscle pains, and genital and urinary complaints [32]. At some point during the session, when some degree of therapeutic alliance has been established, the patient is specifically asked about sexual difficulties and pregnancy-related problems, including past experience of CSA.

The second session is held with the director of the treatment center and the appointed therapist, in order to establish the exact ED and comorbid psychiatric diagnosis. At some point, the therapist emphasizes that "at time, an ED may be conceptualized as a desperate act representing difficulties in coping with adverse life circumstances and stressors and with unexpressed emotional pain". The therapist then proceeds to describe the disorder's multifactorial nature. The patient is encouraged to contemplate about potential triggers for her illness and about specific reasons for seeking help at that time.

If the patient has received treatment previously, she is asked about it, including what was useful and what was less useful for her progress, as well as about her involvement in setting the therapeutic goals and the treatment process. The likelihood of CSA is carefully assessed at this stage. A treatment plan based on all information is then offered, and the patient's feedback to this plan is assessed.

The information gathered, and the patient's reaction to the suggested treatment plan, are indicative of the degree of her future cooperation and the intensity of care required. The team tailors the intervention in line with these indications. If inpatient treatment is required in specifically high risk conditions, the patient receives a detailed explanation of the pros and cons of outpatient versus inpatient treatment with respect to her specific circumstances. The final decision takes into consideration the condition of the patient alongside her need for empowerment and control, from both the patient's and therapist's perspectives.

The Treatment Protocol

Phase I—Evaluation, Immediate Intervention and Stabilization (Around 4 months)

This phase involves evaluation by a multidisciplinary team and psychoeduation about the goals of the treatment, with particular emphasis on the association between CSA and EDs. The immediate treatment goals are to improve the patient's physical condition and reduce her ED symptoms and other health threatening behaviors, including SIBs. As no treatment approaches have been explicitly tailored for young adult patients AN, it is our practice to use dietetic counseling combined with supportive therapy if the ED symptoms are more severe, and psychodynamic psychotherapy with dietetic counseling in patients with less severe ED symptomatology. This is also our practice in adolescent patients with AN, taking into consideration the inherent problems with family therapy in the context of potential CSA. CBT or DBT may be suggested in patients with B/P symptomatology. In the case of severe mood and behavior dysregulation, and/or high risk of self-harm, attempted suicide and re-victimization, DBT may be more effective than other therapeutic interventions, at least in the short run. CBT is indicated mainly if ED-related B/P symptoms prevail. Medications are administered as required. Parents in all types of EDs are requested to supervise meals and health-threatening behaviors. This is done only with the patient's consent and if it is established that the parents themselves are not considered to represent a threat. If there is a suspected risk on behalf of the parents, professional mentors and/or significant others not considered to represent a risk for the patient supervise the meals.

Phase II—Working Through (Around 12 months)

This phase involves individual psychodynamic therapy for patients, separate psychodynamic group counseling for parents, and family therapy for the whole family. The separate treatment modules create a therapeutic space for both the patient and her family for the disclosure of CSA. Relative nutritional and physical stability have to be achieved to allow for underlying trauma-related issues to resurface and to be worked through. It is our experience that patients with an ED and a history of CSA may indicate their readiness to begin trauma work once their ED symptoms and other disruptive behaviors have been brought under reasonable control. The aim of the therapeutic process at this stage is to link current mental distress with previous (often early) abuse events that may have brought about body-hatred and self-harm behaviors. Working with sexual trauma is a slow and complex process of putting together fragment after fragment, eventually establishing some degree of mental continuity. The treatment inherently stimulates transference and countertransference issues within the therapeutic process that can be potentially tied with early abuse experiences. This highly complicated process has to be undertaken in the context of a multidisciplinary team specializing in both EDs and CSA.

Phase III—Integration (Around 4 months)

In this phase patients work through previous treatment-elicited material in individual and/or group settings. The group allows for ventilation of transference-related issues invoked in individual psychotherapy. The aim is to terminate treatment when the patients have experienced at least some integration of the traumatic experiences and contents with ED-related and other relevant material, and when achieving a sense of empowerment and effective coping skills. At this stage, patients are expected be able to self-regulate internal and external situations with the skills acquired in the first CBT/DBT phase of the treatment, and with the cognitive and emotional insights achieved in the second phase. They may also be able to alter their maladaptive ED- and trauma-related relations with their body, taking control over their body and reducing behavioral and psychosomatic expressions of distress.

Two different sets of outcomes may be achieved at this phase:

1. Patients who are in advanced stages of physical, symptomatic, and psychological stabilization may be able to terminate treatment.
2. Patients terminating the three therapy stages but continue to show some degree of ED-, comorbid-, and/or trauma-related symptomatology and/or experience emotional and/or behavioral difficulties may proceed with one of the two following group therapy formats.

(a) Group therapy focusing on rehabilitation and enhancement of coping skills.

This group format include participants between the age of 20–30 years with combined ED and trauma history who have undergone long-term, specialized multidisciplinary therapy in our center as described, yet continue to experience some degree of symptomatic maladjustment. In addition, their overall functioning is impaired in at least one area, including school, work, social life or sustaining stable relationships. The group meets weekly for 6 months. Patients may join a second group if the goals of the treatment have not been fully achieved.

(b) Group therapy focusing specifically on the trauma and its consequences.

The format of this group is based on a model developed by Herman [51] to assist victims of CSA with recounting their stories in the presence of witnesses and to work through their experiences to facilitate recovery. The model consists of 12 sessions and has been adapted for ED patients by Gur and Zubery [54]. The first group working with this model has been composed of patients receiving long-term individual psychodynamic psychotherapy, exhibiting relatively minor ED symptoms and self-harm behaviors, but having difficulty in sharing their CSA stories in individual therapy. In its original form, the traumatic experience has been processed in the group while simultaneously continuing with individual therapy. In its present format, group treatment follows the termination of individual therapy.

The premise underlying this model is that some patients experiencing CSA will recover only after being able to "think the unthinkable and speak the unspeakable" (p. 26) [61]. A group setting enables to address the need voiced by Langberg [62]: "What is too terrifying to hold for long moments in the mind must be remembered and reflected upon. That which is utterly impossible to put into words, must finally be spoken about again and again. Not only must the indescribable be described, but that which so powerfully isolates one human being from others must be uttered within the context of relationship if healing is ever to occur" (p. 12).

The group operates simultaneously on two corresponding planes: the content of the traumatic event(s) and the reenactment of the trauma within the group. Patients are encouraged to recount their stories and explore potential differences and similarities between the two planes. They share years-long amnesias and moments of remembrance, reconstructed stories, self-blame, and doubts as to whether the trauma has really occurred. They further voice their body hate and abuse of their body, re-victimization, re-association of dissociated contents, and their relationships with the perpetrators (whether within or outside the family) and their family at large. At the same time, the dynamics in the group sessions may involve reenactment of the trauma, with the facilitators portraying the parents and the other participants portraying the siblings.

Three Case Vignettes

One participant began a group session by stating: "I had intimate relations with my brother from the age of 8 for 4 years. He is 4 years older, but I'm not angry at him". This statement elicited different reactions from the group members. One member, surviving abuse by her grandfather, angrily retorted: "you were *abused* by your brother", thus forcing her own experience and position upon the other member. At the end of the session, the other participants expressed their anger with the facilitators, feeling that the patient who shared her experience was attacked by the other. They stated that participants were not supposed to be attacked in the group forum. The facilitators, in turn, reflected to the participants that despite the actual threat felt in the room, and although they might have felt during the session as unprotected as when experiencing the original trauma, they were not paralyzed as might have been the case in earlier conditions. Instead, the members fended for themselves, demanding their facilitators to stop the abusive event. The facilitators acknowledged the lack of protection felt in the session, assuming responsibility for their share in it and ending the threat. They further considered the possibility that the participants themselves have the ability to offer guidelines for the group, and to take part in establishing its identity. Sharing of ideas and feelings was used instead of self-harm behavior to terminate the "abusive event".

Another participant wrote to the facilitators: "After the first group sessions, it has become increasingly difficult for me to meet my parents. The feeling of being divided is what I find most difficult to deal with. In most of our family meetings, my father acts as if everything is normal. This reinforces that part of me which feels that none of this has really happened, that I am making it up, and that I am a terrible monster for thinking or saying these things about my father. However, there are other times when I do believe that these things have happened, but that I have been responsible for them, again making me a horrible monster. I feel that I do belong in this group (which is something that I have initially feared would not be the case), but on the other hand I feel so different, because the other participants are not responsible for what has happened to them. I am different: I have brought this upon myself. I have so much to say in the group, but the words are hard to utter. Please help me learn to speak…". She has signed her name and added: "I do not relate to this name at all. The man who calls himself my father has chosen it for me." At the end of the group process this woman has been able to tell her story, decreasing her sense of self-blame; she has stopped cutting herself and managed to improve her eating behavior. Although by the end of treatment she has still been unable to part from her parents, she has decided to visit them only once every 2 months and never on her own. Recently, she has confronted her mother. This woman is now in a bitter fight with her father, who tries to exclude her from the family.

The third description is related to material elicited in a group session of another patient with combined ED and trauma history treated for a long time in both an outpatient and inpatient setting. She stated: "Father kept saying things about my breasts and my buttocks. Maybe he was saying it because I was so sick and he wanted me to put on some weight, or maybe I reminded him of my mother when she was younger. As the years went by, I felt that I couldn't be seen whenever he was around, I wanted to disappear…; since then, whenever I thought that someone is looking at my breasts, I went crazy. I wanted to remove my breasts, erase every sign of femininity. It's true that my father had not actually done anything wrong to me; my grandfather did, but my father had hurt me more. I know that my father did love me, but whenever he talked with me he was ambiguous. I don't think he wanted to harm me. My grandfather was also a good man and everyone loved him. He knew something about medicine and used to give everyone massages. The problem was that as I used to suffer from stomachaches, I had to go constantly to my grandfather for treatment…"

"There is something about this which remains unclear to me to this day. My parents used to drive me to my grandfather because of my stomachaches. Slowly I began feeling that something was not right. Nothing is clear to me anymore because even after I had moved to boarding school, I kept visiting my grandfather and grandmother, even though I knew what was going to happen. I felt that it was wrong, but went anyway…"

"My body betrays me. I do not want to experience any bodily sensations anymore. I am sick of my body and tend to get irritated on account of it. I am disgusted with my whole being. I have considered removing my breasts, my stomach, my legs. I even thought that I am a lesbian, but I am not. I used to make myself sick many times a day so that there was no way I would be reminded of anything—that's the way it used to be at least. But lately it doesn't help anymore. Now nothing sits well in my stomach and everything disgusts me. Sometimes I eat and feel the need to lie down and feel the helplessness in lying on top of my stomach with everything disgusting me. I cannot find anything that tastes good anymore. I feel helpless in keeping food inside me and not throwing it up."

Conclusions

It is now recognized that many women suffering from EDs have experienced some form of sexual abuse during their childhood [13]. This requires the therapists to determine whether their patient with an ED has a history of CSA, in the same way that pediatricians are required to test for lead poisoning in children living in high-risk conditions [1]. It is of note that a history of CSA is more prevalent in patients with EDs diagnosed with B/P behaviors than in restricting type EDs. Moreover, B/P behaviors may be conceptualized as a means to alleviate the pain associated with the traumatic event similar to SIBs or to substance abuse [28]. Accordingly, the treatment of patients with coexisting ED and CSA showing B/P pathology may proceed along different lines than the treatment of restrictive type ED patients with a history of CSA.

In our model, we propose different treatment strategies for patients with combined ED and CSA according to the presence or absence of B/P symptoms only in the first symptomatic phase of the treatment. Therapy in the next phases is similar for all types of EDs. This takes into consideration the premises of Fairburn's transdiagnostic model [62] and of Kaye's [63] conceptualizations with respect to the considerable overlap in the vulnerability factors predisposing to and maintaining B/P and restrictive type EDs, despite the different phenomenological presentations of these disorders.

Professionals treating patients with EDs with a history of CSA must have in-depth knowledge, training and expertise about both problems and about many other comorbid disturbances. Although only a few studies have related to the occurrence of false memory syndrome [60] in EDs [64], its likelihood in this population cannot be overlooked because of the ethical and moral dilemmas involved. Nonetheless, it should be noted that this paradigm has not been accepted by the DSM-V or ICD-11 whereas the concept of dissociative amnesia has been accepted by both diagnostic systems.

Still, the treatment of CSA-related material in our model starts only when the patients' physical condition and eating-related symptomatology are stabilized, at least to some extent. Moreover, as our team is familiar with the issue of false memories, we make every effort to refrain from leading questions, relying on the patients' freely reported recollections. This requires a sound therapeutic stance, in which the therapist listens very carefully to the patient, refraining from any direct or indirect suggestion that the patient might have experienced an abuse event. Yet, the therapist will facilitate the patient's recollections, acknowledging the abuse memories as they resurface [34].

The treatment of CSA victims with EDs is a complex endeavor, as it may intensify negative emotions related to the trauma, increasing, in turn, the risk for maladaptive ED-related and other health-threatening behaviors. Furthermore, treating ED symptomatology may put victims of CSA in a position of relinquishing a powerful affective regulation strategy on which they have come to rely, thus intensifying the trauma experience and its consequences, at least in the short run. Herman [51] claims that since the core of a traumatic experience lies in the act of being denied one's power and detached from others, recovery is based on empowerment and the forming of new relations. Therefore, it is assumed that an intervention in which the patient is disempowered might fail. Still, the continuation of ED symptomatology is not only harmful by itself, but on the long run drains the patient's energies rather than empowering her. Accordingly, an intricate interplay between stabilizing the patient's physical condition and ED symptomatology at least to some extent while enabling her empowerment at the same time is an inherent part of the treatment of patients with coexistent EDs and CSA.

To conclude, our integrated model combines the knowledge of experts in both EDs and CSA. At the core of this model is the need to empower the patient by decreasing her social isolation and sense of helplessness and increasing the range of adaptive options for coping with trauma-related issues and achieving an overall sense of control over her life. It assumes that ED symptoms have to be stabilized to some extent, whether in an outpatient or inpatient setting, using individual therapies of different formats or combined individual and group therapy, before trauma-related issues can be effectively worked through. Thereafter, CSA treatment can be applied in individual and/or group format.

We believe that integrated ED-CSA treatment model can benefit patients seeking therapy in either ED or CSA treatment centers. Still, our recommendations are only preliminary as this model has not yet been subjected to systematic research. Randomized control trials must be undertaken to compare our model to other interventions before any definite conclusions may be reached with respect to utility, adverse effects, credibility, acceptance, and the training and expertise required of therapists who are not necessarily experts in both disorders.

Take home points

- A high rate of CSA history is found in patients with EDs, particularly of the B/P subtype.
- Patients with an ED and a history of CSA exhibit often diverse psychiatric comorbidity in addition to the ED, in particular mood, anxiety, somatoform and/or dissociative disorders.

- Patients with coexisting EDs and a history of CSA also exhibit disorders related to impulse dyscontrol and disruptive behaviors (e.g. SIBs, suicidal tendencies, risk-taking behaviors and addictions).
- A history of abuse has been often associated with treatment failure in patients with an ED if abuse-related issues are not addressed at least to some extent.
- Our integrated treatment model has the advantage of combining the knowledge of experts in both EDs and CSA.
- At the core of the model is the need to empower the patient.
- Treatment of abuse may intensify negative emotions related to the trauma, increasing the risk for maladaptive ED-related and other health-threatening behaviors, at least in the short run.
- Treating abuse-related issues can take place only when some degree of physical rehabilitation and symptomatic stabilization has been achieved and some anxiety-reduction skills have been acquired, At this point, the patients may become more able to work through their emotional and cognitive trauma-related information.
- Patients and family are treated separately
- Integrated ED-CSA treatment can benefit patients seeking therapy in either ED or CSA treatment centers.

Acknowledgments The authors wish to thank Dr. Anat Gur for her major contribution over the years to our awareness of the extent of CSA history among patients with an ED and for sharing her vast clinical experience.

References

1. Wooley SC. Sexual abuse and eating disorders: The concealed debate. In: Fallon P, Katzman MA, Wooley SC, editors. Feminist perspectives on eating disorders. New York: Guilford Press; 1994. p. 171–211.
2. Kearney Cook A, Striegel-Moore RH. Treatment of childhood sexual abuse in anorexia nervosa and bulimia nervosa: A feminist psychodynamic approach. Int J Eat Disord. 1994;15:305–19.
3. Miller KJ. Prevalence and process of disclosure of childhood sexual abuse among eating disordered women. In: Schwartz MF, Cohn L, editors. Sexual abuse and eating disorders. Bristol, PA: Brunner/Mazel Inc; 1996. p. 36–51.
4. Fallon P, Wonderlich SA. Sexual abuse and other forms of trauma. In: Garner DM, Garfinkel PE, editors. Handbook of treatment for eating disorders. New York: Guilford Press; 1997. p. 394–414.
5. Brewerton TD. Bulimia in children and adolescents. Child Adolesc Psychiatr Clin N Am. 2002;11:237–56.
6. Brewerton TD. Eating disorders, victimization and co morbidity: principles of treatment. In: Brewerton TD, editor. Clinical handbook of eating disorders: An integrated approach. New York: Marcel Dekker Inc; 2004. p. 509–45.
7. Brewerton TD. Psychological trauma and eating disorders. Eat Disord Rev. 2005;1:137–54.

8. Brewerton TD. Co morbid anxiety and depression and the role of trauma in children and adolescents with eating disorders. In: Jaffa T, McDermott B, editors. Eating disorders in children and adolescents. Cambridge, UK: Cambridge University Press; 2006. p. 158–68.
9. Brewerton TD. Eating disorders, trauma, and comorbidity: focus on PTSD. Eat Disord. 2007;15:285–304.
10. Jacobi C, Hayward C, De Zwaan M, Kraemer H, Agras WS. Coming to terms with risk factors for eating disorders: application of risk terminology and suggestions for a general taxonomy. Psychol Bull. 2004;130:19–65.
11. Jacobi C, Morris L, De Zwaan M. An overview of risk factors for anorexia nervosa, bulimia nervosa, and binge eating disorder. In: Brewerton TD, editor. Clinical handbook of eating disorders: An integrated approach. New York: Marcel Dekker Inc; 2004. p. 117–63.
12. Smolak L, Murnen SK. A meta-analytic examination of the relationship between child sexual abuse and eating disorders. Int J Eat Disord. 2002;31:136–50.
13. Wonderlich SA, Brewerton TD, Jocic Z, Dansky BS, Abbott DW. The relationship of childhood sexual abuse and eating disorders: a review. J Am Acad Child Adolesc Psychiatry. 1997;36:1107–15.
14. Connor K, Davidson J. A brief global assessment of post-traumatic stress disorder. Int Clin Psychopharmacol. 2001;16:279–84.
15. Vanderlinden J, Vandereycken W. Trauma, dissociation, and impulse dyscontrol in eating disorders. Bristol, PA: Brunner/Mazel; 1997.
16. Yackobovitch-Gavan M, Golan M, Valevski A, Kreitler S, Bachar E, Lieblich A, et al. An integrative quantitative model of factors influencing the course of anorexia nervosa over time. Int J Eat Disord. 2009;42:306–17.
17. Grilo CM, Masheb R. Childhood psychological, physical, and sexual maltreatment in outpatients with binge eating disorder: frequency and associations with gender, obesity, and eating-related psychopathology. Obes Res. 2001;9:320–5.
18. Striegel-Moore RH, Dohm FA, Pike KM, Wilfley DE, Fairburn CG. Abuse, bullying, and discrimination as risk factors for binge eating disorder. Am J Psychiatry. 2002;159:1902–7.
19. Jaite C, Schneider N, Hilbert A, Pfeiffer E, Lehmkuhl U, Salbach-Andrae H. Etiological role of childhood emotional trauma and neglect in adolescent anorexia nervosa: a cross-sectional questionnaire analysis. Psychopathology. 2012;45:61–6.
20. Johnson JG, Cohen P, Kasen S, Brook JS. Childhood adversities associated with risk for eating disorders or weight problems during adolescence or early adulthood. Am J Psychiatry. 2002;159:394–400.
21. Rind B, Tromovitch P, Bauserman R. A meta-analytic examination of assumed properties of child sexual abuse using college samples. Psychol Bull. 1998;124:22–53.
22. Groth-Marnat G, Mitchell K. Responsiveness to direct versus indirect hypnotic procedures: the role of resistance as a predictor variable. Int J Clin Exp Hypn. 1998;46:324–33.
23. Brady KT, Killeen TK, Brewerton TD, Lucerini S. Comorbidity of psychiatric disorders and posttraumatic stress disorder. J Clin Psychiatry. 2000;61S:22–32.
24. Woodside BD, Staab R. Management of psychiatric comorbidity in anorexia nervosa and bulimia nervosa. CNS Drugs. 2006;20:655–63.
25. Levitt JL. Treating eating disorder patients who have had traumatic experiences: a self-regulatory approach. Eat Disord. 2007;15:359–72.
26. Neumark-Sztainer D, Story M, Hannan PJ, Beuhring T, Resnick MD. Disordered eating among adolescents: associations with sexual/physical abuse and other familial/ psychosocial factors. Int J Eat Disord. 2000;28:249–58.
27. Van der Kolk BA, McFarlane AC. The black hole of trauma. In: Van der Kolk BA, McFarlane AC, Weiaeth L, editors. Traumatic stress: the effects of overwhelming experience on mind, body, and society. New York: Guilford Press; 1996. p. 3–23.
28. Steinberg S, Tobin D, Johnson C. The role of bulimic behaviors in affect regulation: different functions for different patient subgroups? Int J Eat Disord. 1990;9:51–5.
29. American Psychiatric Association. Diagnostic and statistical manual of mental disorders. 4th ed. Washington, DC: Author; 1994.

30. Spiegel D, Cardena E. Disintegrate experience: the dissociative disorders revised. J Abnorm Psychol. 1991;100:366–78.
31. Pettinati HM, Horne RL, Staats JM. Hypnotizability in patients with anorexia nervosa and bulimia. Arch Gen Psychiatry. 1985;42:1014–6.
32. Courtois CA. Healing the incest wound: adult survivors in therapy. New York: WW. Norton; 1988.
33. Kessler RC, Sonnega A, Bromet E, Hughes M, Nelson CB. Posttraumatic stress disorder in the National Co-morbidity Survey. Arch Gen Psychiatry. 1995;52:1048–60.
34. Courtois CA. Complex trauma, complex reactions: assessment and treatment. Psychother Theory Res Pract. 2004;41:412–25.
35. Ballenger JC, Davidson JR, Lecrubier Y, Nutt DJ, Foa EB, Kessler RC, et al. Consensus statement on posttraumatic stress disorder from the International Consensus Group on Depression and Anxiety. J Clin Psychiatry. 2000;61S:60–6.
36. Foa E, Rothbaum B. Treating the trauma of rape: cognitive-behavioral therapy for PTSD. New York: Guilford Press; 2001.
37. Keane T, Foa E, Friedman M. Effective treatments for PTSD: practice guidelines from the international society for traumatic stress studies. New York: Guilford Press; 2000.
38. Foa EB, Davidson JRT, Frances A. The expert consensus guidelines series: treatment of posttraumatic stress disorder. J Clin Psychiatry. 1999;60S:6–76.
39. Rothbaum BO, Astin MC, Marsteller F. Prolonged exposure versus eye movement desensitization and reprocessing (EMDR) for PTSD rape victims. J Trauma Stress. 2005;18:607–16.
40. Van der Kolk BA, Spinazzola J, Blaustein ME, Hopper JW, Hopper EK, Korn DL, et al. A randomized clinical trial of eye movement desensitization and reprocessing (EMDR), fluoxetine, and pill placebo in the treatment of posttraumatic stress disorder: treatment effects and long-term maintenance. J Clin Psychiatry. 2007;68:37–46.
41. Marcus MD, Levine MD. Use of dialectical behavior therapy in the eating disorders. In: Brewerton TD, editor. Clinical handbook of eating disorders: an integrated approach. New York: Marcel Dekker; 2004. p. 473–88.
42. Ross CA, Ellason JW. Discriminating among diagnostic categories using the Dissociative Disorders Interview Schedule. Psychol Rep. 2005;96:445–53.
43. Becker CB, Zayfert C. Integrating DBT-based techniques and concepts to facilitate exposure treatment for PTSD. Cogn Behav Pract. 2001;8:107–22.
44. Bradley RG, Follingstad DR. Group therapy for incarcerated women who experienced interpersonal violence: a pilot study. J Trauma Stress. 2003;16:337–40.
45. Allen JG. Coping with trauma. A guide to self-understanding. Washington, D.C.: American Psychiatric Press; 1995.
46. Levitt JL. A self-regulatory approach to the treatment of eating disorders and self-injury. In: Levitt JL, Sansone RA, Cohn L, editors. Self-harm behavior and eating disorders: dynamics, assessment and treatment. New York: Brunner-Routledge; 2004. p. 211–28.
47. Levitt JL, Sansone RA, Cohn L, editors. Self-harm behavior and eating disorders: dynamics, assessment and treatment. New York: Brunner-Routledge; 2004.
48. Levitt JL. A self-regulation treatment approach for the patient with an eating disorder and borderline personality disorder. In: Sansone RA, Levitt JL, editors. Eating disorders and personality disorders: exploring the frontier. New York: Brunner-Routledge; 2006. p. 183–96.
49. Persons JB. Empiricism, mechanism, and the practice of cognitive- behavior therapy. Behav Ther. 2005;36:107–18.
50. Zayfert C, Becker CB. Cognitive behavioral therapy for PTSD: a case formulation approach. New York: Guilford Press; 2007.
51. Herman JL. Trauma and recovery. New York: Basic Books; 1992.
52. Pelcovitz D, Der Van, Kolk BA, Roth S, Mandel F, Kaplan S, Resick P. Development of a criteria set and a structured interview for disorders of extreme stress. J Trauma Stress. 1997;10:3–16.

53. Zeligman Z, Solomon Z. Critical and clinical perspectives on incest. Israel: Hakibutz Hameuchad Publishing House Ltd; 2004.
54. Gur A, Zubery E. Child Sexual Abuse and eating disorders—treatment perspectives. Sexual abuse in the family. The Association of Rape Crisis Centers in Israel. 2010:30–4.
55. Steele K, van der Hart O, Nijenhuis ERS. Phase-oriented treatment of structural dissociation in complex traumatization: Overcoming trauma-related phobias. J Trauma Dissociation. 2005;6:11–53.
56. Zubery E, Binsted N, Zifman N, Jeczmien P. Family therapy model. Adolescents resisting treatment: Exploring the resistance in eating disorder patients to treatment within the family system. Israel J Psychiatry Relat Sci. 2005;42:146–53.
57. Zubery E, Stein D, Latzer Y. Family based program focused on parents (FB-FT) in outpatient care: cognitive behavioral methods combined with a psychodynamic approach in group settings. In: Sassaroly S, Ruggerio GM, editors. The Cognitive model of eating disorders on control, perfectionism, worry and metacognition. New York: Nova Publishers; 2010. p. 131–48.
58. Lock J, Le Grange D, Agras WS, Moye A, Bryson SW, Jo B. Randomized clinical trial comparing family-based treatment with adolescent-focused individual therapy for adolescents with anorexia nervosa. Arch of Gen Psychiatry. 2010;67:1025–32.
59. le Grange D, Crosby RD, Rathouz PJ, Leventhal BL. A randomized controlled comparison of family-based treatment and supportive psychotherapy for adolescent bulimia nervosa. Arch Gen Psychiatry. 2007;64:1049–56.
60. Loftus EF. The repressed memory controversy. Am Psychol. 1994;49:443–5.
61. Bion WR. Experiences in groups. London: Tavistock; 1961.
62. Langberg DL. Counselling survivors of sexual abuse. Wheaton, Illinois: Tyndale; 1997.
63. Fairburn CG, Cooper Z, Shafran R. Cognitive behavior therapy for eating disorders: A "transdiagnostic" theory and treatment. Behav Res Ther. 2003;41:509–28.
64. Jacoby GE, Braks K, Köpp W. Reports on sexual abuse by eating-disordered women before and after psychotherapy: a comparison of anamnestic and catamnestic data. Eur Eat Disord Rev. 1997;5:171–83.

Chapter 9
Interpersonal Maintaining Factors in Eating Disorder: Skill Sharing Interventions for Carers

Janet Treasure and Gill Todd

Abstract The aim of this paper is to describe an intervention designed to share information and skills with carers of people with an eating disorder. The NICE guidelines recommend outpatient management as the first line of treatment for all forms of eating disorders. Hence family members are called upon to provide support within the community. However they are often at a loss as to how best to help. It is common for carers to become anxious, depressed, discouraged and lonely. This can color judgment and some reactions to eating disorder symptoms can be harmful rather than helpful. In both naturalistic studies and randomized controlled trials, family factors have been implicated either as moderators or mediators of outcome. For example high expressed emotion (criticism, hostility and over protection) can adversely impact on the illness. Families can inadvertently be drawn in by the nature of the illness to adjust and accommodate their lives around the symptoms or even enable the continuation of some symptoms. Carers recognize their need for information about how to manage the problem. Sharing information and skills with family members can correct some of the unhelpful attributions and reactions to the illness and can empower non-professional carers to contribute to the process of treatment.

Introduction

In this paper we discuss the theoretical rationale for involving family members in the treatment of people with eating disorders. Firstly we discuss carer's needs. Secondly, we summarise the evidence that suggests that interpersonal processes within the family can act to maintain the illness. Finally we discuss how to share information and skills with carers of people with an eating disorder in order to empower them to be active members of the treatment team.

J. Treasure (✉) · G. Todd
Section of Eating Disorders, Institute of Psychiatry, Psychology & Neuroscience, King's College London, 103 Denmark Hill, London SE5 8AF, UK
e-mail: janet.treasure@kcl.ac.uk

Y. Latzer and D. Stein (eds.), *Bio-Psycho-Social Contributions to Understanding Eating Disorders*, DOI 10.1007/978-3-319-32742-6_9

Family members are eager to help the person with an eating disorder get over their illness but recognize that they are lacking information about what to do [1]. Uncertainties about the causes, course and cures for eating disorders means that there is no clear coherent illness model, which makes the process of information sharing difficult [2]. This lack of information combined with symptoms that produce an overt disruption of eating, a basic core function of living, produces a variety of negative emotions [3, 4]. These color the interpersonal context. High levels of anxiety, for example, are associated with over protection (a component of high expressed emotion), whereas frustration and lack of skills in managing the difficult behaviors are linked to criticism (the other key component of high expressed emotion [5].

Unmet Carers' Needs

Families are usually involved in the treatment of adolescents. However the transition between child and adolescent and adult services involves an abrupt change in the treatment ethos. Carers have reported that they have needs for information and support that are not met by health services. Family members are often excluded by adult services. This is either because the person with an eating disorder is not ready to change and so has not fully engaged in treatment or because health professionals are reluctant to include the families often citing confidentiality as the reason. Thus carers' needs regularly go unmet in adult settings and the treatment context excludes a valuable resource. In this paper we describe an approach that can allow carers of people with all forms of eating disorder and at all stages of the illness and life to join in treatment.

The Key Role of Maintaining Factors in Planning Treatment of an Eating Disorder

Treatments for eating disorders have often been adapted from those designed for other conditions such as depression. Developing tailored treatment to specifically target those factors that either act to cause or maintain symptoms may produce a better fit. Many of the risk factors that we are confident about are fixed and difficult or impossible to change (gender, obstetric trauma etc.). However maintenance factors, those variables that predict symptom persistence over time among initially symptomatic individuals can be modified by specific treatment interventions. We summarise what is known about the interpersonal factors that maintain eating disorders in the following section.

Interpersonal and Family Maintaining Factors

Social factors have been commonly found to adversely affect outcome in people with eating disorders. Steinhausen [6] reviewed the literature on factors relevant for the outcome of anorexia nervosa (data from over 5000 patients with varying follow-up lengths between 1 and 29 years were included) and Fichter and Quadflieg [7] produced a comprehensive review of the outcome of bulimia nervosa (data from 2860 patients followed for between 1 and 12 years). Bulik and colleagues have recently updated this literature [8].

Family factors in particular were highlighted as key prognostic factors in the Australian and New Zealand guidelines [9]: good outcome is associated with minimal weight loss (BMI >17 kg/m^2), absence of medical complications, strong motivation to change behavior, and supportive family and friends who do not condone the abnormal behavior. The variables that predict a poor outcome include: degree of weight loss, long duration of illness, vomiting in emaciated patients, onset in adulthood, co-existing psychiatric or personality disorder, and disturbed family relationships. Thus in addition to features that describe clinical severity and comorbidity (which in most studies of anorexia nervosa includes obsessive compulsive traits) the relationship with the family is of particular importance. Families with more difficulties and individuals with more compulsive traits did better with a more extensive course of treatment (family therapy) [10].

A Model Describing How Interpersonal Factors Interact with Eating Symptoms

Schmidt and Treasure have detailed a four factor model to explain the maintenance of anorexia nervosa [11]. Two dispositions that precede the onset may be both causal and maintaining risk factors. These are compulsive traits, rigidity and perfectionism and high anxiety and avoidance. The other two are consequences of the symptoms, i.e. starvation and disturbed eating habits, which cause close others to respond with reactions of high expressed emotion (overprotection and criticism) and the biological and psychological changes which are perceived to be positive for the individual. It is beyond the scope of this article to describe all the evidence supporting this model but we will briefly summaries what is known about interpersonal/family factors illustrated in Fig. 9.1. These are of key importance for the information and skill sharing interventions that we describe here.

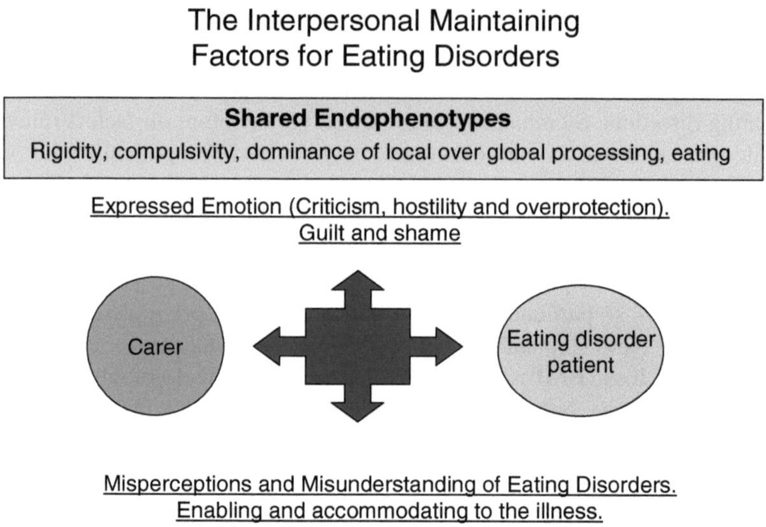

Fig. 9.1 A model illustrating the shared vulnerability and interpersonal factors that maintain eating disorders. This figure outlines the shared endophenotype relating to dispositions for emotional avoidance, obsessive compulsive traits and eating behaviors and the emotional, cognitive and behavioral consequences that can arise in the presence of eating disorder shared vulnerabilities

The Endophenotype Conceptualization

The first two maintaining factors, compulsivity and high anxiety, within the four factor model, "Valued and Visible", precede the onset of eating disorders. It is possible that these are endophenotypes associated with the genetic underpinning of eating disorders (for a detailed account of endophenotypes and phenotypes see the following reviews) [12–15]. It follows from this endophenotype, genetic conceptualization of eating disorders that family members will also share these characteristics. Thus all first degree family members may also be prone to anxiety, rigidity and compulsivity. Also other family members may have their own eating issues. There is evidence to support this proposition. Family studies have found that first degree relatives have higher levels of obsessive compulsive personality disorders [16], eating disorders and obsessive compulsive traits. Thus the high anxiety and distress reported by carers of people with eating disorders [3] may not arise merely from the stress caused as a consequence of living with a relative with an eating disorder, but may result from an interaction between a difficult situation and a sensitive disposition. These traits may shape the response to eating disorder symptoms.

Interpersonal Interactions

A variety of emotions, thoughts and behavioral factors shape the interpersonal reactions that result when a family member has an eating disorder. These include the following:

1. Rigidity, compulsivity, preoccupation with detail.
2. Expressed emotion (criticism, hostility and overprotection).
3. Guilt and shame.
4. Misperceptions and misunderstanding of eating disorders.
5. Enabling and accommodating to the illness.
6. Avoidance of emotions.

Rigidity, Compulsivity, Preoccupation with Detail

Carers share some of these traits with the individual with an eating disorder. Such traits can interfere with effective problem solving and therefore make it difficult to flexibly adapt for a change in family function. Rigidity and compulsivity do not promote thinking which generates new ways of behaving. It is interesting that Minuchin's clinical conceptualization of anorexia nervosa as a paradigm of psychosomatic families included rigidity as a relevant construct [17]. The difficulty in stepping back to see the bigger picture is often associated with an overly analytical focus and can mean that carers join in a dialogue with some of the anorexia nervosa rules. This merely serves to validate and reinforce them. This inflexibility makes for difficulty in problem solving. The inability to step back and focus on the big picture means everyone may fight over details. By such means these traits can underpin some of the accommodating and enabling behaviors.

Expressed Emotion (Criticism, Hostility and Overprotection)

Criticism, hostility and overprotection are the components of expressed emotion that have been associated with poor outcome in a variety of psychiatric illnesses [18]. Carers of people with eating disorders have high levels of expressed emotion. In a study which compared parents of people with eating disorders with parents of young people living at home over 60 % (96/151) of carers showed high emotional over-involvement (EOI) compared to 3 % (3/93) of controls [5]. This level of over protection was noteworthy as the people with anorexia nervosa were older (aged 23 years) than the comparison group (aged 17 years). It had proved difficult to obtain an age matched comparison group with young people at home, as in the UK the majority of people matched to the educational attainments of the group with anorexia nervosa left home for college or university at 18 years. Over protection was associated with high levels of anxiety. The level of criticism was three times higher in the carers of people with eating disorders 47 % (71/151) compared to 15 % (14/93) of the carers in the comparison group. Criticism was associated with difficult behaviors.

Several studies have found that expressed emotion (EE) affects adherence to treatment and/or outcome in AN [19–25]. Thus reducing family levels of expressed emotion may improve the prognosis of anorexia nervosa. Indeed family based interventions are associated with a reduction in expressed emotion [24–26].

Interestingly, there is also the suggestion that the level of expressed emotion can moderate the impact of treatment. For example, families with high expressed emotion have a better outcome with separated family therapy (where the parents are seen separately from the patient) rather than conjoint family therapy [21]. More recently in a study of interventions for adolescent bulimia nervosa the outcome was better if carers with high expressed emotion were involved in a family based intervention than if guided Cognitive Behavioral Therapy (CBT) was used [27].

Overall, there is preliminary evidence from a small but consistent body of work that suggests that the type of close interpersonal interaction captured in the construct of expressed emotion may be a causal maintaining factor in an eating disorder. This effect is probably most pronounced where there are high levels of contact between the person with an eating disorder and their carers. This is most relevant to young adolescents and to more severely ill patients who are not able to live independently.

Guilt, Shame and Stigma

The concept of expressed emotion does not capture guilt, shame and stigma, commonly found in carers of people with eating disorders [4]. In part these emotional reactions can arise because there is recognition that traits shared in common may have caused the eating disorder. For example, this feature is highly characteristic of parents with their own eating problems. The stigma associated with not being able to feed a child and the label of a mental illness both contribute to a sense of failure in carers. The dependency of the individual with the eating disorder and stigma associated with the illness were highly predictive of carers' distress [2].

Misperceptions and Misunderstanding of Eating Disorders

The lack of a clear, coherent, conceptualization of eating disorders can contribute to difficult interactions in the family. In a qualitative study of the experience of caring for people with anorexia nervosa we found that misperceptions about the illness were linked to criticism and hostility [4]. Terror about the consequences led to an over protective style of interacting with accommodation to, and even acceptance of, some of the symptomatic behaviors [4]. In the early phase of the illness negative appraisals about care giving were common alongside the worry that there would be severe consequences. Another less positive appraisal of care giving was associated with the belief that the illness was attributable to the sufferers' personality [2]. These emotional reactions may lead to avoidance and social isolation which in turn can increase the distress and shelter the eating disorder from normalizing influences [28].

Enabling and Accommodating to the Illness

Family members can reinforce eating disorder symptoms with a variety of accommodating and enabling behaviors. These are behaviors whereby the family are positively reinforcing or removing any negative consequences of the eating disorder. This can include the family allowing eating disorders symptoms to dominate the house hold: accepting and even pandering to eating disorder rules (where, why, how, when and with whom, etc.) relating to: food and eating, safety behaviors (exercise, vomiting, body checking, fasting or cutting back), obsessive-compulsive behaviors (reassurance seeking, counting, checking and control). This acceptance of eating disorder related behavior is forced upon families by explicit or implicit emotional black mail or threatening behavior by the patient. For example, if eating disorder rules are disobeyed then the patient may not eat at all or will harm herself or act destructively in other ways. In addition the individual with an eating disorder may compete, compare or calibrate her/himself with other family members (often siblings) in terms of what and how much to eat or exercise. Again this behavior is tolerated in an effort to keep the peace and because there is fear about resisting because of "Edi's" fragile state. Finally family members may be drawn into enabling the eating disorders by covering up, or removing or buffering the natural negative consequences that would accrue from the behavior e.g. replacing missing food, cleaning kitchen and bathroom, making excuses to others etc. The assessment of families includes a functional analysis of typical interpersonal interactions to reveal and define these unhelpful patterns of behavior [29].

Avoidance of Emotions

Avoidance of emotions can also be a dispositional trait not associated with high expressed emotion, where the emotional management model in the home is on a continuum where the polar opposites are over control or under control of emotions. The eating disorder provides a mechanism by which the sufferer manages their emotions through the disorder so that all emotions are numbed. Emotional regulation is not learned and self-compassion or compassion for others is missing or directed to the exhausting effort of attempting to please others at all costs.

The Developmental History of Information and Skill Sharing Interventions

It is beyond the scope of this article to go into detail about the variety of forms of family treatments that have been used to treat people with eating disorders and more specifically in anorexia nervosa. The "Maudsley model" of family therapy, an early intervention approach for adolescents with a short duration of illness has been mannualized and has now been used in a range of treatment studies [30]. Meanwhile the form of family work has been modified and has included: separated family therapy (parents seen in parallel to the adolescent [21]); multifamily groups of various configurations either including the offspring [31–34] or not [24].

This treatment modality has now been adapted to fit the needs of carers of treatment resistant cases of anorexia nervosa and bulimia nervosa and for use in a variety of different modes of delivery. In particular we have distilled the essence of what is required to manage the challenge of eating symptoms into a form that can be shared with family members and also used as a training tool for clinicians.

Evolving from an iterative process of research and development we have developed a variety of methods of sharing information and skills with carers of people with eating disorders including a manual, DVDs, workshops, telephone coaching, etc. The aim is to address carer's needs and also to interrupt some of the maintaining mechanisms defined both in our theoretical model [11] and our research into the experiences of family members [35, 36]. In the initial phase of this work developed over 10 years ago we explored the use of this approach for carers of people with the treatment resistant form of anorexia nervosa i.e. inpatients in our specialist unit [37]. The content has since been modified on the basis of the qualitative and quantitative feedback from both patients and their carers involved in that study and used in the context of carers of a wider patient group.

Aims of the Information and Skill Training Intervention

The overall aim of this intervention is to give carers skills so that they can act as a coach to help and support the person with an eating disorder in her journey of recovery. Essentially we offer carers a short course in the management of eating disorders. This is similar in content to courses we offer specialist health professionals. We start with a discussion of "transference" issues but this is translated into the form of animal metaphors to make it easy to understand and to inject humor and lightness into the proceedings. We give carers information about how to improve their own coping strategies to reduce burnout and stress. Next we teach skills on how to side step reacting with any of the means of maintenance described above. The process of training includes theories such as the principles of the trans theoretical model of change and functional analysis and skills such as better communication using the principles of motivational interviewing and problem solving [4].

Table 9.1 Description of maintaining factors associated with the intervention's target

Interventions targeted at maintaining factors	
(1) Rigidity, compulsivity, preoccupation with detail, eating	Education and feedback. Remediation to ameliorate extreme traits
(2) Expressed emotion (criticism, hostility and overprotection)	Education and discussion about "transference" issues. Training in role modeling issues
(3) Guilt and shame	Education about illness. Role-plays. Contact with other carers
(4) Misperceptions and misunderstanding of eating disorders	Education about illness. Group discussions. Contact with other carers
(5) Enabling and accommodating to the illness	Functional analysis. Training in communication
(6) Emotional avoidance	Education, discussion and feedback. Remediation to recognize and ameliorate this trait

Initially these principles are applied by carers to themselves as they learn to change their own relationship with the eating disorder. Next, we teach carers how to implement these skills to help their relative with an eating disorder change their behavior. The teaching can be done in groups, 1:1, via telephone coaching and is currently being developed to be delivered as an online distance learning package.

A summary of how the intervention is used to target maintaining factors is shown in Table 9.1.

Results of Information and Skill Sharing Interventions

The initial study of this skills training intervention, was in the form of family day workshops on an inpatient unit. We found that the new intervention was equivalent to a standard form of individual family therapy in terms of the outcome for patients and for carers. The qualitative feedback from the carers was positive in that they particularly enjoyed the structured skills training [38]. This encouraged us to develop the intervention further. The second phase of our research involved running training workshops consisting of six 2-h sessions to supplement the skills based manual. The results from the pilot study were encouraging enough to continue with a randomized trial [35]. This form of intervention was acceptable to carers, satisfaction was high and carer's feedback was positive. The content and structure of the workshops were also judged to be relevant and useful. The level of distress and caregiving difficulties especially in those who were living with the relative was decreased. These changes were maintained over a 3-month period. However, when we compared the workshops to a waiting list, we did not observe any beneficial effect in terms of carer stress level [39]. Many carers were unable to access the workshop resource due to problems with time or distance. We therefore developed a training program digital video-technology format based upon educational content of the workshops. This program was presented on five DVDs. The Manual and DVDs were supported with telephone coaching. The pilot results from this intervention using DVDs as training tools suggested that parents found it to be helpful and acceptable [36]. An advanced study with the DVDs shows promising results [40].

Common Concerns About Skills Sharing with Families

Some carers are somewhat skeptical and reluctant to be involved in family work [41], but we have found that the information and skill sharing format is more acceptable. Interventions with some face to face contact such as the workshop can defuse some of the guilt and stigma and allow the opportunity for interpersonal learning and guided practice. Issues of privacy and confidentiality with fears about intrusions into family life are less marked with this type of intervention as individual patients are not discussed by the group facilitators.

We have found that people with eating disorders themselves are sometimes reluctant for carers to have contact with professionals. This could be because they fear that their carer may become more skilled in fighting the anorexia nervosa or bulimia nervosa. One of the first steps that carers may need to take in order to become more effective is to make a stand about their rights and their entitlement to go and get help and support for themselves.

Conclusions

Automatic and understandable reactions to eating disorder behaviors can inadvertently act to reinforce the symptoms. A variety of factors can contribute to these effects including: shared vulnerability traits relating to compulsions, eating and an over analytical focus; misappraisals about the causes of the illness and the pathways to cure; over protection and or criticism (expressed emotion) and guilt and shame; accommodating and enabling behaviors.

Carers lack information and skills to manage eating disorders but are highly motivated to contribute to treatment. Information and skills training interventions focused on these maintaining factors hold promise as methods of producing effective early interventions and reduce the burden and distress of managing treatment resistant cases. Eating is a family affair and so are eating disorders.

Take home points

- Eating is a family affair and so are eating disorders.
- Carers lack information and skills to manage EDs but are highly motivated to contribute to treatment.
- Automatic and understandable reactions to ED behaviors can inadvertently act to reinforce the patients' symptoms and distress.

- A variety of factors can contribute to these reactions of family members, including: shared vulnerability traits relating to compulsions, eating, an over analytical focus and a lack of self-compassion; misappraisals about the causes of the illness and the pathways to cure; over protection and or criticism (expressed emotion) and guilt and shame; and accommodating and enabling behaviors.
- Information and skills training interventions focused on these maintaining factors hold promise as methods of producing effective early interventions and reduce the burden and distress of managing and living with treatment resistant cases.

References

1. Haigh R, Treasure J. Investigating the needs of carers in the area of eating disorders: development of the Carers' Needs Assessment Measure (CaNAM). Eur Eat Disord Rev. 2003;11:125–41.
2. Whitney J, Haigh R, Weinman J, Treasure J. Caring for people with Eating Disorders: factors associated with psychological distress and negative caregiving appraisals in carers of people with eating disorders. Br J Clin Psychol. 2007;46:413–28.
3. Treasure J, Murphy T, Szmukler G, Todd G, Gavan K, Joyce J. The experience of caregiving for severe mental illness: a comparison between anorexia nervosa and psychosis. Soc Psychiatry Psychiatr Epidemiol. 2001;36:343–7.
4. Whitney J, Murray J, Gavan K, Todd G, Whitaker W, Treasure J. Experience of caring for someone with anorexia nervosa: qualitative study. Br J Psychiatry. 2005;187:444–59. doi:10.1192/bjp.187.5.444.
5. Kyriacou O, Treasure J, Schmidt U. Expressed Emotion in Eating Disorders assessed via self-report: an examination of factors associated with Expressed Emotion in carers of people with Anorexia Nervosa in comparison to control families. Int J Eat Disord. 2008;41:37–46.
6. Steinhausen HC. The outcome of anorexia nervosa in the 20th century. Am J Psychiatry. 2002;159:1284–93.
7. Fichter MM, Quadflieg N. Six-year course of bulimia nervosa. Int J Eat Disord. 1997;22:361–84.
8. Berkman ND, Lohr KN, Bulik C. Outcomes of eating disorders: a systematic review of the literature. Int J Eat Disord. 2007;40:293–309.
9. Beumont PJV, Hay P, Beumont D, Birmingham L, Derham H, Jordan A, et al. Australian and New Zealand clinical practice guidelines for the treatment of anorexia nervosa. Aust N Z J Psychiatry. 2004;38:659–70.
10. Lock J, Agras WS, Bryson S, Kraemer HC. A comparison of short- and long-term family therapy for adolescent anorexia nervosa. J Am Acad Child Adolesc Psychiatry. 2005;44:632–9.
11. Schmidt U, Treasure J. Anorexia nervosa: valued and visible. A cognitive-interpersonal maintenance model and its implications for research and practice. Br J Clin Psychol. 2006;45:1–25.
12. Steiger H, Bruce K. Phenotypes, endophenotypes and genotypes in bulimia-spectrum eating disorders. Can J Psychiatry. 2007;52:220–7.
13. Steiger H. Eating disorder paradigms for the new millennium: do "attachment" and "culture" appear on brain and genome scans. Can J Psychiatry. 2007;52:209–11.
14. Treasure J. Getting beneath the phenotype of anorexia nervosa: the search for viable endophenotypes and genotypes. Can J Psychiatry. 2007;52:212–9.

15. Bulik C, Hebebrand J, Keski-Rahkonen A, Klump KL, Reichborn-Kjennerud T, Mazzeo SE, et al. Genetic epidemiology, endophenotypes, and eating disorder classification. Int J Eat Disord. 2007;40(Suppl):S52–60.
16. Lilenfeld LR, Kaye WH, Greeno CG, Merikangas KR, Plotnicov K, Pollice C, et al. A controlled family study of anorexia nervosa and bulimia nervosa: psychiatric disorders in first-degree relatives and effects of proband comorbidity. Arch Gen Psychiatry. 1998;55: 603–10.
17. Minuchin S, Baker L, Rosman BL, Liebman R, Milman L, Todd TC. A conceptual model of psychosomatic illness in children. Family organization and family therapy. Arch Gen Psychiatry. 1975;32:1031–8.
18. Butzlaff RL, Hooley JM. Expressed emotion and psychiatric relapse: a meta-analysis. Arch Gen Psychiatry. 1998;55(6):547–52.
19. Eisler I, Szmukler GI, Dare C. Systematic observation and clinical insight-are they compatible? An experiment in recognizing family interactions. Psychol Med. 1985;15:173–88.
20. Eisler I, Dare C, Russell GF, Szmukler G, Le Grange D, Dodge E. Family and individual therapy in anorexia nervosa. A 5-year follow-up. Arch Gen Psychiatry. 1997;54:1025–30.
21. Eisler I, Dare C, Hodes M, Russell G, Dodge E, Le Grange D. Family therapy for adolescent anorexia nervosa: the results of a controlled comparison of two family interventions. J Child Psychol Psychiatry. 2000;41:727–36.
22. Szmukler GI, Eisler I, Russell GFM, Dare C. Anorexia nervosa, parental 'expressed emotion' and dropping out of treatment. Br J Psychiatry. 1985;147:265–71.
23. Szmukler GI, Berkowitz R, Eisler I, Leff J, Dare C. Expressed emotion in individual and family settings: a comparative study. Br J Psychiatry. 1987;151:174–8.
24. Uehara T, Kawashima Y, Goto M, Tasaki SI, Someya T. Psychoeducation for the families of patients with eating disorders and changes in expressed emotion: a preliminary study. Compr Psychiatry. 2001;42;132–8.
25. van Furth EF, van Strien DC, Martina LM, van Son MJ, Hendrickx JJ, van Engeland H. Expressed emotion and the prediction of outcome in adolescent eating disorders. Int J Eat Disord. 1996;20:19–31.
26. Eisler I, le Grange D, Asen E. Family Interventions. In: Treasure J, Schmidt U, van Furth EF, editors. Handbook of eating disorders. 2nd ed. Chichester: Wiley; 2003. p. 291–311.
27. Schmidt U, Lee S, Beecham J, Perkins S, Treasure J, Yi I, Eisler I. A randomized controlled trial of family therapy and cognitive behavior therapy guided self-care for adolescents with bulimia nervosa and related disorders. Am J Psychiatry. 2007;164(4):591–8. doi:10.1176/appi.ajp.164.4.591.
28. Sepulveda AR, Whitney J, Hankins M, Treasure J. Development and validation of an eating disorders symptom impact scale (EDSIS) for carers of people with eating disorders. Health Qual Life Outcomes. 2008;6:28.
29. Hibbs R, Rhind C, Sallis H, Goddard E, Raenker S, Aytonc A, et al. Confirmatory factor analysis for two questionnaires of caregiving in eating disorders. Health Psychol Behav Med. 2014;2:322–34.
30. Lock J, Le Grange D, Agras WS, Dare C. Treatment manual for anorexia nervosa. A family based approach. New York: Guilford; 2001.
31. Dare C, Eisler I. A multi-family group day treatment programme for adolescent eating disorder. Eur Eat Disord Rev. 2000;8:4–18.
32. Colahan M, Robinson PH. Multi-family groups in the treatment of young adults with eating disorders. J Fam Ther. 2002;24:17–30.
33. Geist R, Heinmaa M, Stephens D, Davis R, Katzman DK. Comparison of family therapy and family group psychoeducation in adolescents with anorexia nervosa. Can J Psychiatry. 2000;45:173–8.
34. Scholz M, Aser E. Multiple family therapy with eating disordered adolescents: concepts and preliminary results. Eur Eat Disord Rev. 2001;9:33–42.

35. Sepulveda AR, Lopez C, Todd G, Whitaker W, Treasure J. An examination of the impact of Maudsley eating disorder collaborative care workshops on the well being of family members. Soc Psychiatry Psychiatr Epidemiol. 2008;43:584–91.
36. Sepulveda AR, Lopez C, MacDonald P, Treasure J. Feasibility and acceptability of DVD-based skills training for parents of people with an eating disorder. Int J Eat Disord. 2008;41:318–25.
37. Whitney J, Murphy T, Landau S, Gavan K, Todd G, Whitaker W, et al. A practical comparison of two types of family intervention: an exploratory RCT of family day workshops and individual family work as a supplement to inpatient care for adults with anorexia nervosa. Eur Eat Disord Rev. 2012;20:142–50.
38. Treasure J. Anorexia nervosa. A survival guide for sufferers and those caring for someone with an eating disorder. Hove: Psychol Press; 1997.
39. Whitney J, Currin L, Murray J, Treasure J. Family work in Anorexia Nervosa: a qualitative study of carers' experiences of two methods of family intervention. Eur Eat Disord Rev. 2012;20:132–41.
40. Sepulveda AR, Todd G, Whitaker W, Grover M, Stahl D, Treasure J. An exploratory randomised trial of a support programme for carers of patients with eating disorders. Int J Eat Disord. 2010;43:603–10.
41. Whitney J, Eisler I. Theoretical and empirical models around caring for someone with an eating disorder: the reorganization of family life and inter-personal maintenance factors. J Ment Health. 2005;14:575–85.

Part III
Sociocultural Issues

Chapter 10
Emotional First Aid in Eating Disorders: The Unique Role of Hotlines and Online Services

Itzhak Gilat and Yael Latzer

Abstract Over the last five decades, volunteer-based hotlines and online services have become an attractive source of emotional first aid. This chapter examines the unique role that these services play for individuals who suffer from eating disorders (ED), particularly anorexia nervosa and bulimia nervosa. The theoretical advantages of hotlines and online services for ED clients are presented, stressing the fact that they exact a lower psychological price from the clients than professional sources of help. The therapeutic potential of these services for ED patients is demonstrated by means of empirical studies on the characteristics of calls to the hotlines, and the analyses of two online interactions representing two types of assistance that hotlines and online services offer ED patients: paving the way to professional therapy for those who shy away from it, and offering patients who do undergo treatment a supportive environment. The evidence leads to the conclusion that the role played by hotlines and online services complements professional sources.

Introduction

Eating disorders, especially Anorexia Nervosa (AN) and Bulimia Nervosa (BN), are severe diseases that may lead to destructive consequences. If they remain untreated, the lives of the individuals who suffer from them are at risk high mortality and

I. Gilat (✉)
Levinsky College for Education, Tel Aviv, Israel
e-mail: gilati@netvision.net.il

I. Gilat
Head of Online Services in the Israeli Association for Emotional First Aid (ERAN), Netanya, Israel

Y. Latzer
Faculty of Social Welfare and Health Sciences, Haifa University, Mount Carmel, Haifa, Israel

Y. Latzer
Eating Disorders Institute, Rambam Medical Center, Haifa, Israel

Y. Latzer and D. Stein (eds.), *Bio-Psycho-Social Contributions to Understanding Eating Disorders*, DOI 10.1007/978-3-319-32742-6_10

morbidity and poor prognosis. A major component of AN and BN is a subjective experience of acute emotional distress that markedly impairs quality of life and may trigger suicidal behavior. It is reasonable to assume that patients with AN or BN would be anxious to seek professional help in order to reduce the risk and alleviate the pain. However, the abundant clinical and empirical evidence points to the contrary. Patients who suffer from eating disorders—anorexics in particular—exhibit low willingness to seek treatment [1, 2]. Several explanations have been suggested for this maladaptive attitude, including perceiving the symptoms as beneficial, reducing cognitive dissonance by adopting the belief that they have chosen the symptoms, or protecting themselves against the threat of an alternative identity [3]. These causes may be conceptualized in terms of the "psychological price" that acts as a barrier to seeking help [4].

Even when they commence treatment, patients with anorexia nervosa frequently demonstrate resistance, refuse to cooperate with the therapist, and sabotage the chances for an effective outcome [1]. A pattern of enduring resistance may engender a countertransference response from the therapist and further jeopardize the success of the therapy. For instance, one study found that therapists felt less connected and engaged and more frustrated with anorexic and bulimic patients than with clients with depression [5].

It might be concluded that the inability of Eating Disorders (ED) patients to benefit from the professional help that is so indispensable to them is attributable to two barriers: they perceive the "psychological price" of the therapy as too high, and they elicit a negative attitude from their therapists. One strategy for coping with these barriers is to develop special helping agencies that meet two conditions: first, to reduce the psychological price of the interaction with the helper, and second, to alter the disruptive interpersonal processes between the ED patient and her helpers and generate a help-promoting environment. A volunteer-based telephone counseling service (hotline) can be viewed as an appropriate agency for this purpose owing to its unique features, as shown in the next section.

Characteristics of Volunteer-Based Hotlines

Hotlines were developed in the 1950s for the purpose of crisis intervention and suicide prevention, and became an attractive source of emotional first aid in a wide spectrum of domains [6]. The literature cites several features of hotlines that explain their popularity as a community-based source of psychological help [1, 6, 7]. Client anonymity: The option of retaining anonymity creates an emotionally safe environment that encourages openness and self-disclosure. Anonymity may be particularly vital with respect to problems that evoke an emotional threat such as sexual abuse [2]. Helper anonymity: Since the volunteer remains anonymous and unseen, the caller may shape the character of the helper according to his/her needs. This situation promotes positive transference that may be helpful for an individual in distress who may be avoiding confronting a real helper [3]. Client control: Unlike face-to-face encounters, where the therapist wields most of the power, the client remains in his/her space, visual cues regarding the therapist's status are eliminated, and the caller can terminate the interaction whenever he/she chooses [4]. Use of paraprofessionals: The use of trained volunteers is guided by the rationale that they may successfully use the requisite skills—such as warmth and empathy to offer emotional first aid to individuals in crisis [8]. Volunteers may evoke less threat as compared to professionals since the context of the helping interaction is perceived as more humanistic than therapeutic [5]. High accessibility: Since assistance is available 24 h a day, individuals can receive help when the need arises. In addition, the elimination of space barriers enables callers to receive help regardless of their location and physical limitations.

Volunteer-based emotional first aid services were expanded to the online environment soon after the Internet became a major player in the communications arena. Some of the features that made the telephone an attractive source of emotional help are also characteristic of the online environment and may even exert a more powerful effect on the extent of the caller's openness. The anonymity that prevails in the online environment is almost complete and has been shown to significantly increase emotional expressions in interpersonal communication. This phenomenon has been entitled the "disinhibition effect" [9]. The fact that the helper's ambiguity is greater online than it is on the telephone promotes the projection and facilitates positive transference.

A unique characteristic of the Internet that may enhance the success of helping interactions is text-based communication. Empirical evidence suggests that a text environment affords emotional protection against the therapist's negative reactions, such as criticism and boredom, and increases self-disclosure [9, 10]. In addition, it shows that writing enhances therapeutic processes [11]. Another unique advantage of the Internet is the variety of available patterns of communication. Individuals who seek psychological help may receive relevant information on a non-interactive web page, participate in an online support group (either synchronous or asynchronous), opt for a one-on-one real-time conversation through personal chat, or send an email. This variety of options enables them to choose the source that is most appropriate for them.

The advantages of the hotlines and the online volunteer-based services for ED patients are demonstrated in the next section by the empirical and clinical evidence gathered by the Israeli Association for Emotional First Aid (ERAN), a community-based mental health service that offers both telephone and online assistance. The distressed clients are responded to by volunteers who are trained and supervised by a team of mental health professionals. The first branch of ERAN was established in Jerusalem and began to operate there in 1971. Over the years, ERAN became a nationwide mental health service offering emotional support and crisis intervention by telephone to the general population. In 2002, ERAN expanded its services to the Internet and provided emotional first aid by means of online support groups, personal chats, and email. For a review see [12].

Calls to ERAN from Individuals Who Suffer from Eating Disorders: Empirical Evidence

The theoretical considerations presented above suggest that telephone hotlines may be uniquely suited to providing psychological assistance to individuals suffering from eating disorders. An epidemiological survey on calls to ERAN was conducted in order to test this assumption [13]. More specifically, the study sought to examine the frequency of calls regarding eating disorders and to compare the portraits of the callers to those of callers presenting other mental problems.

The study was conducted during the years 1994–1997. During this time, ERAN had 500 volunteers who operated in eight branches all over the country and responded to about 50,000 calls per year. The study data comprised 19,776 calls, constituting a representative sample of all the calls that were received in ERAN during that period. The instrument for gathering the data was a structured form that the volunteers routinely completed at the end of each call. The following variables were measured by the form: (1) age and sex of the caller; (2) type of call (new/recurrent); (3) history of professional treatment (present/absent); (4) caller's expectations, defined by two categories that were not mutually exclusive: emotional support (present/absent) and practical advice (present/absent); (5) main problem presented by the caller. The volunteers identified the main problem from a list of specific problems that was defined on the basis of a content analysis of calls to ERAN. These problems were grouped into six major categories: intra-personal, interpersonal, family, sexuality, environmental pressures (i.e., work-related stress), and mental disorders. ED is one of the specific problems in the category of mental disorders, which also includes psychosis, anxiety, post-traumatic- stress- disorder, depression, substance abuse, and "other" disorders.

To assess the prevalence of ED calls to ERAN, two measures were computed: (1) Prevalence of ED calls among the total number of calls to ERAN. This measure was computed by the number of calls in which ED was defined as the main problem out of the total number of calls received by ERAN. (2) Prevalence of ED calls among calls presenting mental disorders. This measure was computed by the number of calls in which ED was defined as the main problem out of the total number of calls in which mental disorders were defined as the primary problem.

The prevalence of ED among the total population of calls was found to be related to the sex and age group of the caller. While very few ED calls were received from males, ED constituted 0.4 % of the calls from adult females and 2 % of the calls from adolescent females. An examination of the prevalence of ED among female adolescents as a function of time revealed a steady increase. The percentages were 1.0, 1.7, 2.1 and 3.1 for the years 1994–1997, respectively.

The prevalence of ED among calls presenting mental disorders revealed different patterns for adult and adolescent females. Only one percent of the calls from adults were focused on ED, while psychoses (47 %), depression (22 %), and anxiety (19 %) constituting the major categories. In the case of adolescents, ED was the second most frequent problem, identified in 18 % of the calls, with anxiety being the most frequent (26 %), and depression (16 %) the third most frequent.

In order to examine the characteristics of ED calls, this group was compared to the group comprising other psychological disorders in three dimensions: type of call, history of professional treatment, and caller's expectations. The analyses yielded the following results: (1) The percentage of new callers was significantly higher among ED (63 %) than other mental disorders (22 %). (2) Receiving emotional support from the volunteer occurred less frequently as the main expectation among ED callers (62 %) than among callers with other disorders (86 %), whereas receiving practical advice was more frequently expected by ED callers (61 %) than by callers with other mental disorders (20 %). (3) ED callers received psychological treatment (58 %) significantly more frequently than callers with other mental disorders (40 %).

The systematic increase in the proportion of adolescent girls with ED who sought help from ERAN suggests that the hotline may be viewed by many such individuals as an appropriate source of help. The appeal of hotlines for young women with ED is further illustrated by the finding that ED problems were the second most frequently occurring of all the psychological disorders presented by adolescent girls. It is interesting to note that anxiety-related problems were the most frequent, and depression was almost as common as ED calls. Since affective and anxiety disorders are often comorbid among women with ED [14], it is reasonable to assume that many requests for help concerning anxiety or depression may mask ED-related problems. Hence, the actual proportion of ED callers to the hotline may be even higher than that indicated by the number of calls directly defined as ED.

With regard to the nature of the help sought by the ED callers, it was found that about 60 % of them had applied for professional therapy before calling the hotline, while the remaining 40 % used the hotline as their first formal source of help. These two groups of callers may represent two types of expectations from the hotline. The non-patient callers probably decided to make the first move in their effort to relieve their mental distress in the framework of the emotionally safe environment afforded by the telephone hotline. The function of the hotline for this category of ED callers is to facilitate a smoother entry into professional therapy. This function is consistent with the recommendation that resistance to treatment be viewed as an evolutionary process whereby initial refusal is gradually transformed into recognition of the advantages of the therapy [1]. Patient-callers probably call the hotline to work through feelings of frustration that emerge in the therapy process and focus on their relationship with the therapist. Such feelings may arise from the resistance to treatment that is characteristic of ED patients.

The epidemiological study described above focused on the analysis of ED calls to the hotline as an entire group, and did not distinguish among the subcategories of ED. In order to examine whether the hotline plays a differential role for different subgroups of eating disorders, a comparative analysis was conducted to examine the help-seeking characteristics of four subcategories of ED: AN, BN, Binge Eating

Disorder (BED) and Eating Disorder-Not Otherwise Specified (ED-NOS) [15]. The data consisted of 147 calls received by the Israeli hotline from individuals suffering from an ED. Ninety percent of the callers were women. The distribution of calls according to age-group revealed that 21 % were received from adolescents, 23 % from young adults (19–25 years old) and 56 % from adults. Data were gathered by means of the same standard form employed in the epidemiological study described above. However, the present study also utilized the open-ended section of the form where a detailed description of the conversation is reported by the volunteer.

Results revealed that of the ED calls to the hotline, 32 % were directly related to AN, 28 % to BN, 25 % to BED, and 15 % to other eating disorders (ED-NOS). The diagnostic categories of ED were examined in relation to the identity of the caller, i.e., whether the caller was the individual suffering from ED or a significant other associated with the ED patient, such as a family member or a friend. The results revealed that calls from significant others were significantly higher among AN (46.5 %) and BN (40.5 %) than among BED (3 %) and ED-NOS (10 %). This finding may reflect the ambiguity and helplessness experienced by people involved with AN and BN patients as well as their own pressing need for help as a result of the guilt and shame characteristic of significant others and their reactions to these diseases [16].

The four diagnostic categories were compared with regard to three help-seeking characteristics: type of caller (new vs. recurrent), type of expectation from the call, and referral for treatment. The results revealed that BED callers differed from the AN, BN, and ED-NOS callers with respect to all three characteristics. BED callers were characterized by a higher frequency of recurrent callers (73 %), while the other three categories comprised mainly new callers (84, 74, and 73 % for AN, BN, and ED-NOS, respectively); BED callers expected emotional support rather than instrumental help, while the opposite was true of the other callers; the percentage of callers referred to professional treatment was very low among BED callers (6 %), moderate among AN and BN (30 % each), and relatively high among ED-NOS callers (56 %).

The results suggest that BED and AN/BN callers differ in respect to the type of help they expect to receive from calling the hotline. Most of the callers who suffer from BED are recurrent callers who mainly seek continuous emotional support that may facilitate psychological maintenance. This pattern is characteristic of non-ED callers, such as individuals who suffer from chronic states of depression, anxiety, or schizophrenia. With regard to the AN and BN clients, most of them are first-time callers whose goals are more therapeutic than those of the BED callers. Some of them call the hotline when the process of denial begins to unravel, but confusion, shame, and reluctance to seek professional treatment remain. Others may be undergoing professional treatment but call the hotline in order to process difficulties they encounter in their relationship with the therapist. Thus, the link between the hotline and the professional treatment is complementary—the encounter with the empathetic volunteer smoothes the path to therapy or helps to preserve/maintain this process.

Personal Internet Chats

Utilizing a statistical view of help-seeking characteristics, the two studies presented in the previous section demonstrated the unique role played by hotlines in assisting individuals suffering from ED. By analyzing two personal chats, the next section focuses on the interpersonal process that occurs between the ED client and the volunteer. Personal chats are synchronous (real-time) conversations between two participants who exchange written texts on the Internet using one of the available types of software such as ICQ. The two chats represent different types of help-seeking among ED clients—paving the way for seeking professional help in the first chat, and providing support and empowerment in the second.

In the first chat, the client was a 23-year-old woman with a history of AN who had a very brief and disappointing experience with professional help from a social worker during her military service. She was afraid of a relapse in her illness, but felt confusion and shame about seeking help. The interaction with the volunteers aimed to pave the way to professional therapy.

Parts of the transcripts are presented below. All identifying details have been totally excluded and minor changes have been made in the story told by the client so as to ensure complete anonymity.

The first chat: I need help but I don't know what to do about it

ERAN: Good evening. What would you like to talk about?

Client: I'm not crazy and I don't intend to commit suicide, but I need help and I don't know what to do about it and who to turn to.

ERAN: You've made the first move and I thank you for this.

Client: And the second move…

ERAN: Most of the people who call us are not crazy and don't want to commit suicide…they just need someone to talk to about something. I'd be glad if you told me.

Client: There are people who love me, but I'm very introverted and don't talk to anyone about my problems.

ERAN: Do you feel that it's hard to talk about certain things with people who are close to you?

Client: It's hard to talk about myself and about my problems.

ERAN: Why is it so difficult for you?

Client: Because I don't think they can help me and I'm ashamed to tell them that I need professional help.

ERAN: Try to tell me first and maybe it'll be easier later.

In this initial phase of the chat, the client displays an unresolved conflict between the need to reduce her distress and the perceived barriers to receive professional help. The volunteer employs various strategies in order to create an atmosphere of trust and support: She reinforces the client's first step to seek help, normalizes her request for help, and encourages her to disclose her feelings and thoughts in the environment of the chat.

Client: There are various things that I'm carrying with me from childhood. I hate the way I look and I don't succeed in the things I do.

ERAN: Give me an example of something you hate about the way you look.

Client: I'm tired of maintaining the proper weight and trying to lose weight each time I gain. … I've suffered from eating disorders for a long time, but I've managed to overcome them.

ERAN: Wow…It isn't easy at all. How did you manage to do it?

Client: It's really very difficult. I know that it's really dangerous, but I'd like to be there (thin) again because I looked really good.

ERAN: How thin were you then?

In the following part of the chat, the client described her anorexic symptoms, which were very characteristic of the disorder, and relates that although she felt that she had lost too much weight, she did not manage to gain weight.

Client: When my health problems worsened, I decided to take control of my life.

ERAN: You made a great move. You know that it's very difficult to overcome anorexia; most girls don't succeed.

Client: Thank you. My problem is that even though I know how dangerous it is, I want to be there (thin). I just can't get it out of my mind. It's something I can't explain.

ERAN: I know what you're talking about…It seems to the others around you that everything is all right, but you know from within that it isn't.

Client: Exactly! What you just said is exactly how I feel. Eating isn't the only thing that bothers me. People see me nice and smiling and they have no idea what I'm feeling inside.

ERAN: How much energy is needed to hide all this?

It seems that the volunteer succeeded in gaining the client's trust, thereby getting her to disclose the history of her disorder, the subjective experience associated with it, and the emerging, unfulfilled wish to receive help. The volunteer responds with a combination of empowering the client's strengths as evidenced in her struggle against the disorder, as well as her empathetic attitude toward the client's present state. The client expands her self-disclosure by sharing with the volunteer her painful experience of duality between her internal and external image. This confession causes the volunteer to extend the dialogue into the client's self- perception in the next part of the chat.

ERAN: May I ask what you do in life.

Client: I rent an apartment, study, and work.

ERAN: In spite of all the difficulties. And at the beginning of our chat you said that you don't succeed at anything.

Client: I really don't succeed at anything…

ERAN: You study, you work, you live by yourself, you cope with an ED.

Client: The fact that I study doesn't mean that I succeed. I just know that I cope with all the stresses all alone and it will explode sometime, I live by myself so that my mother won't see my condition, and I study so that my family will think I'm normal like everyone else.

At this point in the conversation, the volunteer decides to shift the focus to the issue of professional help. It seems appropriate in light of the openness and cooperative approach displayed by the client in the course of their conversation.

ERAN: Have you ever undergone any kind of treatment?

Client: During my military service, I saw a mental health officer. I did it because I really wanted help and not in order to be discharged. But I didn't seek any other help because I was ashamed.

ERAN: Did you feel that it helped you?

Client: It did not really help me. In the army they think you're making everything up.

ERAN: Yet you said it helped you a little. It seems to me that you are able to extract the maximum from every situation.

What would you think about calling an ED clinic? It's covered by your medical insurance and you don't have to tell anyone about it.

Client: And nobody will tell my parents about it?

ERAN: No, they won't. You're not a minor.

In any case you can set up an appointment and ask about anything you want to know. The therapist will explain the procedure to you..

Client: I guess I'll do it.

ERAN: It may take some time, and in the meantime don't hesitate to call us when your soul is heavy.

I want to thank you and reinforce you for making this important decision.

Client: Thanks for listening to me.

ERAN: I know it's not easy.

Client: No, it isn't.

ERAN: I wish you success.

Client: Thank you.

Due to the single-session intervention applied in ERAN, we cannot know whether the young client actually did set up an appointment at an ED clinic. However, an examination of this chat within the context of ERAN indicates that it can be deemed effective in light of the client's agreement to seek professional therapy.

The second chat: Let's see how you cope with eating disorders

The client in the second chat is a 17-year-old girl who suffers from AN with a history of hospitalization, who is treated by a psychologist but still experiences an acute state of mental pain with suicidal ideations. The aim of the interaction with the volunteer is to provide a supportive environment boost her self-esteem, and empower her.

In the initial part of the chat, the girl tells the volunteers about her relationship with her boyfriend, who is the only person in the whole world she trusts. Her warm relationship does not prevent her from "sinking into [her] problems". She feels guilty about her preoccupation with her problems while her boyfriend is in the army, fighting a war.

Client: I feel so selfish that I dare to complain while he is stuck over there.

ERAN: You are not selfish at all. It's your right to cope with your problems. They are probably very troubling. At least free yourself from guilt.

Client: I feel so guilty. Three weeks ago I was released from an eating disorder unit at the hospital…I believed it was all behind me, but soon after I came home everything burst out. I have nightmares, I hardly sleep, I feel exhausted, I feel dizzy,faint, drink smoke and I don't know what to do with myself.

ERAN: Did they release you because you felt better?

Client: They released me from the hospital because I thought I was OK…On the other hand I knew that when I got out of hospital I would fall again…but they believed me…I did not deceive them intentionally. I hospitalized myself voluntarily because I really wanted to be healthy, but it is probably more difficult than I thought… Soon I'll be underweight, but I'm so fat…It sounds funny but it's true. In sum, the hospital didn't help at all.

The anorexic girl's monologue expresses the unbearable pain and helplessness that emerged due to the continuous influence of the disorder and the unsuccessful outcome of the most effective weapon—hospital. Her conclusion is common among AN patients:

Client: I feel like I'm breaking down…I'd consider it a favor to everyone if I didn't wake up again. I'm so miserable and I'm sick of coping with everything…

ERAN: What about your parents?

Client: My father doesn't live with us and my relationship with my mother isn't good.

ERAN: You wrote that you're seeing a psychologist. Does he help you? What about friends? I guess it's impossible to cope with this situation alone.

Client: My psychologist is very nice…Friends—friendship is something very loose…I told you that I don't count on people; they will betray me in any case. When I think about it, if I die, everyone will forget about me within a month and no one will suffer, selfish as it may sound, I won't suffer either.

The combination of the severe painful experience caused by the anorexia with the lack of emotional support) is potentially lethal. Her decision to seek help from ERAN can be viewed as an indication of the will to live and may reduce the risk of suicide. The option of chatting online anonymously with a caring volunteer who has not let her down is probably the most appropriate means of receiving emotional support.

ERAN: I can understand that since your pain is so strong, disappearing seems to be an appropriate solution for you. I think that in your condition you can't see what I can see from the outside, but I see that you'll lose many things; one of them is your relationship with your friend. I know it is so painful now, but it is possible to get out of your situation.

Client: It's impossible…impossible…I'm collapsing. My poor boyfriend is an angel. What does he need a dumb, ugly, filthy, repulsive, anorexic girlfriend like me for? I believe that there is nothing good about me. I'm just trash from the street. I'll be doing him a favor.

ERAN: I believe that right now you see yourself that way, but I don't believe this is really you. If an angel like your friend loves you, it means that he sees the wonderful parts of you that you are unable to see at this moment.

Client: You're all living in "a movie!" (an Israeli slang for unrealistic world). I want to die, I need to die. Do me a favor and say OK! Why is it so difficult? Why should I suffer, why? I know I'm trash, but it's unbearable, I'm sick of it!

ERAN: You will not succeed in convincing me that you're trash. You're a girl who needs help; you can improve your condition and be free. Try to think of yourself in a different way. You can become healthy and enjoy life, you have a friend who loves you, there are many years ahead of you—believe me, it's possible!!

Client: Let's see how you'd cope with eating disorders! Hearing voices in your head telling you that you're trash, that you don't deserve anything, that you aren't allowed, that you have no right, that you're a waste, that you're scum, you're stupid, you have no ability, no brains, you're shit! Garbage! A devil! Because this is what goes on in my mind all day long; and even when I look at food, I immediately hurt myself in some way to punish myself for daring to think that I deserve a piece of bread…

It is interesting to note the discourse of this dramatic outburst directed at the volunteer. Although the client is talking about herself, she uses the pronoun "you" in all the negative descriptions, as if she were projecting all of her self-aggression on the volunteer.

Client: I'm sorry, I'm sorry I got mad at with you I'm sorry, I'm really sorry…

ERAN: I wasn't offended, don't worry. I don't suffer from eating disorders, but I know how difficult it is. I've met some anorexic girls and I know that it's like hell. But I also know that you can get out of it and I really hope you succeed.

I'm at the end of my shift. I really wish you that you could get back to normal life, and of course I hope your boyfriend comes home soon.

Client: Thank you, really thank you… Have a good night ☹

The client's gratitude at the end of the chat may indicate that the volunteer's empathy and acceptance were helpful to her in some way. It is reasonable to assume that this supportive environment succeeded in calming her down, albeit temporarily, and may even have prevented a deterioration in her mental state. Her positive experience with this online chat may encourage her to avail herself of this source of emotional first aid in subsequent events of acute crisis.

Conclusion

The original aim of hotlines was to help individuals in suicidal crisis. However, owing to their characteristics, they became an appealing source of help for other groups of distressed people who experienced difficulty in seeking help from conventional sources. The evidence presented in this chapter shows that hotlines and online services constitute a valuable source of assistance for individuals suffering from eating disorders. Theoretically, two explanations may be suggested for the unique contribution of the hotlines. First, they offer conditions such as anonymity and client control that lower the psychological price that deters many ED patients from seeking professional therapy. Second, they enable the ED callers to produce an emotionally supportive environment that decreases counter-transference and promotes an effective relationship between them and their helpers. More specifically, our data indicate two types of help that ED clients can receive from the volunteers: (1) facilitating the first step along the path to professional therapy, and (2) providing emotional support. The first type may be useful for those who recognize the need for help but eschew contact with professionals, and the second type is prevalent among ED patients who are undergoing treatment but need an additional supportive environment in which they can share the feelings and thoughts that arise in their interaction with the therapist. In both cases, the role of the hotlines complements that of the professional agents. Further study is required in order to examine the effectiveness of hotline and online volunteer-based services for individuals who suffer from eating disorders.

Take home points

- The original aim of hotlines is to assist individuals during suicidal crisis.
- Hotline may become an appealing source of help for other groups of distressed individuals experiencing difficulties in seeking help from conventional sources.
- Hotlines and online services may constitute a valuable source of assistance for EDs.
- Hotlines offer conditions such as anonymity and client control that lower the psychological price detering many ED patients from seeking professional therapy.
- Hotlines enable EDs callers to produce an emotionally supportive environment likely decreasing counter-transference issues and promoting an effective relationship with their helpers.
- ED callers can receive support and encouragement from the volunteers to make the first step along the path to professional therapy.
- The role of the hotlines complements that of the professional agents.

References

1. Goldner EM, Birmingham CL, Smye V. Addressing treatment refusal in anorexia nervosa: clinical, ethical and legal issues. In: Garner DM, Garfinkel PE, editors. Handbook of treatment for eating disorders. New York, NY: Guilford Press; 1997. pp. 450–61.
2. Latzer Y, Shatz S. Comprehensive community prevention of disturbed attitude to weight control: a three level intervention program. Eating disorders: Treat Prev. 1999;7:3–31.
3. Yager J. Special problems in managing eating disorders. New York, NY: American Psychiatry Press; 1992.

4. Nadler A. Help-seeking behavior: psychological costs and instrumental benefits. In: Clark MS, editor. Review of personality and social psychology. Newbury Park, CA: Sage; 1992. pp. 290–311.
5. Franko DL, Rolfe S. Countertransference in the treatment of patients with eating disorders. Psychiatry. 1996;59:108–15.
6. Lester D. Counseling by telephone: an overview. In: Lester D, editor. Crisis intervention and counseling by telephone. Springfield, IL: Charles C Thomas; 2002. pp. 5–21.
7. Rosenbaum A, Calhoun JF. The use of telephone hotlines in crisis intervention: A review. J Commun Psychol. 1977;1997(5):325–38.
8. Knickerbocker DA, McGee RK. Clinical effectiveness of nonprofessional and professional telephone workers in a crisis intervention In D Lester, GW Brockop (Eds.), Crisis intervention and counseling by telephone (pp. 298–309). 1973: Springfield, IL: Charles C Thomas.
9. Suler J. The online disinhibition effect. Cyber Psychology Behavior. 2004;7:321–6.
10. King R, Bambling M, Lloyd C, Gomurra R, Smith S, Reid W, Wegner K. Online counseling: The motives and experiences of young people who choose the Internet instead of face to face or telephone counseling. Couns Psychother Res. 2006;6(3):169–74.
11. Wright J, Chung MC. Mastery or mystery? Therapeutic writing: A review of the literature. Br J Guid Counc. 2001;29:277–91.
12. Gilat I, Shahar G. Suicide prevention by online support groups: An Action Theory-based model of emotional first aid. Arch Suicide Res. 2009;13:52–63.
13. Latzer Y, Gilat I. Calls to the Israeli hotline from individuals who suffer from eating disorders: An epidemiological study. Eat Disord. 2000;8:31–42.
14. Pollice C, Kaye WH, Greeno CG, Weltzin TE. Relationship of depression, anxiety and obsessionality to state of illness to anorexia nervosa. Int J Eat Disord. 1997;21:367–76.
15. Latzer Y, Gilat I. Help seeking characteristics of eating disordered hotline callers: Community based study. J Soc Serv Res. 2005;31:61–76.
16. Vandereycken W, Kog E, Vanderlinden J. The family approach to eating disorders. New York, NY: PMA Publishing Corp; 1989.

Chapter 11
The Characteristics of Pro-Ana Community

Meyran Boniel-Nissim and Yael Latzer

Abstract Pro-Ana are websites that are designed to promote and support Anorexia Nervosa (AN) and other eating disorders. Common features of these websites include forums and chat rooms, tips and tricks, 'thinspirations', as well as links to other Pro-Anorexia websites. One of the most common and disconcerting aspects of these websites is the detailed instructions for initiating and maintaining the illness, AN. Pro-Ana members join a special target-based virtual community in order to encourage one another in losing weight and creating a social environment that does not denounce self-starvation, but rather support and strengthens the disordered behavior. The aim of this chapter is to try to identify the characteristics of the Pro-Ana community, to understand the motivations underlining the engagement in these websites and accordingly to suggest clinical and research implications for therapists and researchers.

Introduction

Eating disorders (ED) are mental and psychological disorders associated with impaired eating behaviors, a distorted body image and an obsession with food, body shape and weight [1]. Many women develop abnormal and unhealthy eating behaviors in order to live up to cultural ideal of thinness. This ideal is both widely and intensively expressed and reinforced through family, social, and culture

M. Boniel-Nissim (✉)
School of Social Sciences and Humanities, Kinneret Academic College, Sea of Galilee, Kinneret, Israel
e-mail: meyranbn@gmail.com
URL: http://www.mbn-psychonet.com/

Y. Latzer
Faculty of Social Welfare and Health Sciences, University of Haifa, Haifa, Israel

Y. Latzer
Eating Disorders Institute, Psychiatric Division, Rambam Health Care Campus, Haifa, Israel

Y. Latzer and D. Stein (eds.), *Bio-Psycho-Social Contributions to Understanding Eating Disorders*, DOI 10.1007/978-3-319-32742-6_11

frameworks. This phenomenon is known to affect various populations, including socioeconomic status, nationality, origin and gender [2, 3].

Although personal and genetic predisposition are needed for the development of eating disorders, mass media in itself has an extensive influence. The socio-cultural perception of beauty is stressed in mass media: in articles on beauty and diet in women's journals; in advertisements for hunger depressants and low-calorie food; and in deliberate negative attitude towards overweight people and gaining weight. Thus, women are exposed from various directions to the myth affirming that beauty, success and self-worth are depending on a thin body [3, 4].

Studies show that there is an influence of mass communication such as written media (newspapers and magazines) and audio communication (movie, television and radio) on the emergence of eating disorders [5–7]. In the past decade, the Internet has become a significant communications network for incorporating viewer channels, advertisements and databases. The network is available to everyone and an attractive tool, therefore special attention should be given to the use of this dimension in the field of eating disorders.

The Internet and Eating Disorders

The Internet serves as an invaluable resource for individuals and provides them with a plethora of information and resources. The Internet constitutes a combination of social interaction and transference of acceptable ideas in mass communication. Therefore, the Internet has the power of greatly influence on its users. Those have an infinite number of possibilities to obtain information and connect to social networks, both familiar and not, positive and negative. As Norris et al. [8] suggest, the Internet provides individuals with access to information on a variety of medical issues, including eating disorders; search on the Internet for "Anorexia Nervosa" reviles an abundance of information that is available.

Obtaining health information on the Internet is popular. A survey taken in the United States in 2005 revealed that nine out of ten respondents are searching the web for health information. There is a significantly rising interest in subjects related to dieting and thinness, 51 % in 2004 as opposed to 44 % in 2002 [9]. Technically, searching for information related to body weight and nutrition through search engines usually generates sites related to dieting. In this case, searching for information on losing weight can reveal, unintentionally, information related to destructive ways to lose weight such as the Pro-Anorexia websites. These websites are designed to promote and support AN. The combination of pressure to lose weight, availability of information on the Internet and the ability to translate theory into practice with fast results, can be dangerous, especially for those who are prone to low self-esteem and are looking for quick solutions [8].

It's important to note that the ability to receive recommendations and ideas on how to lose weight for those suffering from AN is not a result of the Internet. In the past, those who were interested could get information from magazines, autobiographical books of women who suffered from AN, as well as from medical psychiatric and diet literature. Another source was support groups of recovered eating disorder individuals. Even so, the Internet reinforced this phenomenon and expanded the boundaries of the legitimate community for women with eating disorders who are not interested in treatment [10–12].

On the Internet because of the freedom to write and advertize, as well as the lack of editing and enforcement, every message is legitimate. Therefore, freedom of expression does not only characterize the positive side of the Internet, but it is also an effective and powerful mean with a negative effect. In particular, it may have an affect on those who are in the process of forming their identity, seeking answers, or predisposed to mental disorders [13]. This is an important cross-road, especially for a teenager girl who is in the early stages of developing an eating disorder, which is characterized by secretive and reclusive behavior.

The Internet and Adolescents

Adolescence is an age with a series of continuous dramatic transitions and adjustments on the physiological, endocrinal and neural level, as well as the psychological, developmental, mental and cognitive level. At the same time, there are changes in other areas of life, for example, within the social and family environment. Naturally, these changes manifest themselves in the adolescents' eating habits weight and shape concern. Beyond physiological growth and development, the two major objectives during the adolescence phase are independence and identity construction. At this stage, the adolescent is in the process of building his physical, affective and functional foundation in preparation for adulthood. The process presents itself in almost every area of the adolescent's life, with parents on one side and the peer group, with all its demands, on the other. The adolescents need to detach themselves from familiar beliefs and opinions. In addition, they begin to rely less on parents while at the same time deal with the demands that the adolescence period presents in a responsible and independent manner. At a later stage, the construction and formalization of a mature identity occurs. The adolescent is required to be responsible, and to acquire the necessary skills needed to integrate a perception of the world that takes into consideration the future. In addition, the adolescent takes essential steps in order to deal with the adult world. This is reflected in the adolescent's autonomy concerning eating that may lead to ED [14].

Teenagers use the Internet very frequently and find it as a convenient place to connect with their peer group. Furthermore, the Internet is a comfortable arena for clarifying and building one's personal identity [15]. Communication via the Internet, based mainly on text, allows the individual to "project" oneself into cyberspace, express sides of one's personality in an authentic way [16]. The anonymity, invisibility, the non-verbal indications and the absence of eye-to-eye contact, all allow one to quickly reveal oneself with nearly no restraint, a phenomenon known as "Online Disinhibition Effect". Thus, the Internet characteristics allow greater self disclosure, sometimes even faster than face-to-face communication [17]. While the ability to turn directly to others and openly apply to the disordered eating is frightening in the physical world, it is legitimate and easy to fulfill on the Internet. The fear of criticism and judgment of one's lifestyle decreases because of the anonymity and invisibility that characterize the Internet [18].

Fear from prejudice may lead the young girl to turn to more creative ways of getting support and finding a sense of belonging in a virtual community. Turning to the Internet represents a junction; while surfing the web, one can go in a certain direction and find information related to eating disorders and Pro-Ana, while taking another path might present that person with information about treatment and recovery from eating disorders. The average age of participants in Pro-Ana sites is 16.7. Since eating disorders are more prevalent among adolescent girls, it's possible that these sites attract adolescent girls who are at risk of developing eating disorders (ED) [19].

Pro-Ana Community

Pro-Ana websites are Internet sites commonly run by individuals with an eating disorder. On these websites, participants provide nonjudgmental support for other individuals who are currently engaged in an eating disorder and not in recovery [10]. Members of this community relate to EDs as a conscious choice and as a lifestyle, but not as a pathological illness that demands treatment. Research has shown that one of the most permanent characteristics of those suffering from ED and in particular AN is denial that a problem exists. Denial typically accrues throughout the entire course of treatment but is most pronounced in the early stages of the illness and in particular among those with AN. The illness considers being egosyntonic in its manner [20].

Pro-Ana members join a special target-based virtual community in order to encourage one another in losing weight and creating a social environment that does not denounce self-starvation but rather supports and strengthens the disordered behavior [10]. Pro-Ana communities can be found in the Internet under different names, such as: Pro-Ana, ANAMADIM, Pro-Anorexia, Pro-ED (Pro-Eating Disorder), Thinspiration, ED's Friends, Starving for Perfection, Dying to be Thin, Pro-Ana/Mia, and Wannarexice.

There has been a lot of controversy surrounding Pro-Anorexia websites over the past decade. In fact in 2001 an American eating disorder advocacy group, Anorexia Nervosa and Associated Disorders (ANAD) pled with Internet servers such as Yahoo to remove these sites. Four days after their plea, 115 sites were shut down. Many other servers have also removed these websites. Dias [10] notes that it is very difficult to locate Pro-Anorexia websites consistently as many sites are shut down daily. However, new sites also emerge on daily basis. There are those who claim that the rejecting and denouncing attitude had the opposite result. These websites became more attractive and intriguing because of the ban on them [21]. Due to the changing nature of these websites it is difficult to determine the number of Pro-Anorexia sites, but Chesley et al. [19] estimate that there are over 500 Pro-Ana websites. Pro-Ana websites have also been shown to be more organized, comprehensive, visited more often, and more numerous than pro-recovery or professional sites. In their study they found that Pro-Anorexia websites had 34,988 visitors, whereas pro-recovery websites had a mean count of 28,878 visits. A recent study showed that within a period of a year, there were more than half a million visits at Pro-Ana's websites in the Netherlands. Also the number of Pro-Anorexia websites hosted by one single provider increased more than 10-fold [22]. Despite the difficulty in accepting the phenomenon, Pro-Ana websites continue to serve as "self-help" sites for the community members. This perception allows major understanding that rejection and banning of the community does not help in eradicating the eating disorder phenomenon, nor does it diminish its value in the eyes of its members [23].

Today, Pro-Ana communities operate underground in the Internet, which means it is hard to find them in a simple search on the web; some links leads to an empty page; others are built under covert names that hide their purpose. Only those who are in the secret know their way around and can connect these sites [11, 12]. The level of comradeship in the community is high and demands secretiveness and clandestineness. Revealing any information about the community is forbidden. As a result, it is difficult to estimate the number of members in the community [18, 24]. Even so, it is important to note that despite the glamour of belonging to a secret community, the concealment is not easy for members. The need to reveal oneself to close ones that are not part of the community are expressed in Pro-Ana forums, despite the unequivocal demand to avoid any form of exposure since this could lead to misunderstanding, destruction of relationships and distress [10, 18].

Characteristics of Pro-Ana Community

Research on Pro-Ana websites have identified several themes which help us to understand the information that is being disseminated through the Internet as well as why individuals join these sites. Individuals join these sites for support and to have a safe place to discuss their anorexic behaviors free from judgment. However, individuals are also being exposed to themes of weight loss, the idea that they have control over their behavior, their behavior is positive, and that sacrifice and deceit are necessary to achieve weight loss goals. Although there are several hundred Pro-Ana websites, most of them appear to have similar themes and are also formatted in a similar manner.

Mulveen and Hepworth [21] suggested that there's a clear distinction made on the Pro-Ana website between AN, the mental illness, and 'Ana' the lifestyle choice. Members in Pro-Ana use an extreme weight loss method where one chooses to use similar techniques as those employed by individuals with AN. The main things that distinguished these two concepts were the perceived degree of control and the choice that individuals had over eating. 'Ana' is presented as being in control and aware, whereas AN is a mental illness. A comparison between Pro-Ana sites and sites that deal with treating ED shows that Pro-Ana sites attract more Internet users.

Evidently, websites of the Pro-Ana community have similar characteristics. One of the main components is pictures that serve as models of inspiration for thinness for members of the community ("thinspiration"). **Thinspirations** can be triggering photographs of slim celebrities, poems, movies, or anything else that is meant to inspire and sustain the behavior associated with AN [25]. Most of the images of thinness and emaciation posted on these websites are images of celebrities and fashion models. The images often mimic themes of dismemberment or focus solely on one body part, both of which are commonly seen in advertisements. As Dias [10] indicates, if the models and celebrities were not familiar to us, it would be difficult to distinguish between the images of the emaciated and deviant bodies of those with AN and the acceptable and idealized bodies of the models. 92 % of the websites that Norris et al. [8] studied contained "thinspirations". They noted that most often "thinspirations" were in the form of visual images but that motivational quotes and writings were also common. Accordingly, pictures of overweight women are presented in order to arouse rejection, as well as to warn from lapsing into that type of situation [18].

Bardone-Cone and Cass [26] designed an experiment in which nine undergraduate women viewed a Pro-Anorexia website, six undergraduate women viewed a comparison website that focused on body image and female fashion (thinspiration), and nine women viewed a neutral control website about home décor. The authors developed the Pro-Anorexia website based on an extensive Internet search of over 300 existing Pro-Anorexia websites. The only individuals that showed an increase in negative affect were those who viewed the Pro-Anorexia website. Similarly, only those who viewed the Pro-Anorexia website showed a decrease in self-esteem. Women who viewed the Pro-Anorexia website also felt less confident in their ability to achieve their ideal weight. Women who viewed the female fashion and home décor websites did not indicate a change in their perceived weight status or their perceived attractiveness to the opposite sex, whereas those who viewed the Pro-Anorexia websites reported an increase in their perceived weight status and a decrease in their perceived attractiveness. These results suggest that viewing Pro-Anorexia websites has a negative impact on how viewers think and feel about themselves. Unfortunately the small sample size and the non-clinical nature of the sample limit the generalization of these results.

Another characteristic of Pro-Ana websites is the tips and methods ("tips & tricks") for losing weight, deceiving family and friends and, in general, misleading the medical team in case of treatment or hospitalization. In addition, there are calculators of body fat levels and caloric intake, recipes, ways of coping with fasting and more. The information is displayed on the website but also in forums and in personal stories which represent the personal experiences of the community members [10, 18]. Eight of the twelve Pro-Ana sites that Norris et al. [8] analyzed included 'tips and tricks.' The tips posted on these websites varied significantly. For example, the 'tips and tricks' page on the website the member *Anagrrl* discussed the most effective diet drugs and where they could be ordered on the Internet [25]. 'Tips and trick' sections also included the topics of starvation, fasts, and complementary and alternative medicines. Norris et al. [8] found that two-thirds of the Pro-Ana sites contained information specifically on calories. Frequently these websites posted foods that are believed to have a negative caloric intake. The tricks found on these websites frequently included ways to hide weight loss and methods for calorie avoidance. Although some of the websites did warn viewers of the dangers associated with extreme weight loss, others provided potentially dangerous information to viewers with no warnings.

The Pro-Ana community defines itself as a **cult** even though it doesn't have all of the characteristics (like paying money, a charismatic leader, or a real contact). As so it adapted religious metaphors, instructions for a lifestyle in the spirit of the Pro-Ana way of thinking and reference lists for inspiration. Religious metaphors were often present in the forms of the "Ana Psalm", Creed and a list of "Cult Principles". Religious messages often centered on issues of control, starvation, and self-hate. On a few sites, these messages almost appeared cult like. For example, on one particular website, followers were encouraged to make a pact with Ana and sign their name in blood. More personal websites also contained letters from Ana. One website that Norris et al. [8] studied posted a "letter from Ana" which read, "*I expect a lot from you. You are not allowed to eat much… I will expect you to drop your caloric intake and increase your exercise. I will push you to the limit. You must take it because you cannot defy me. Pretty soon, I am with you always*". (p. 445).

Another letter from "Ana" that summons to maintain thinness and execute control of their bodies:

> Allow me to introduce myself. My name, or as I am called by so called "doctors", is Anorexia. Anorexia Nervosa is my full name, but you may call me Ana. Hopefully we can become great partners. In the coming time, I will invest a lot of time in you, and I expect the same from you….Sometimes you will rebel. Hopefully not often though. You will recognize the small rebellious fiber left in your body and will venture down to the dark kitchen….When it is over, you will cling to me again, ask me for advice because you really do not want to get fat. You broke a cardinal rule and ate, and now you want me back. I'll force you into the bathroom, onto your knees, staring into the void of the toilet bowl. Your fingers will be inserted into your throat, and, not without a great deal of pain, your food binge will come up. Over and over this is to be repeated, until you spit up blood and water and you know it is all gone. When you stand up, you will feel dizzy. Don't pass out. Stand up right now. You fat cow you deserve to be in pain!…

A survey of 47 Pro-Ana websites showed that 54 % included **cult principles**, for example, "*I believe in perfection and starvation is way of achieving it*"; 27 % included quotations from "Ana" such as, "*Salvation by losing weight*"; 31 % presented "Ana" rules; 21 % went deeper into describing "Ana" as a cult with principles and edicts, for example,

> I dedicate my life to Ana. She will be with me where ever I go, and will make sure that I do not stray. No one else is important. I am committed to respecting her and causing her to be proud of me.

All the declarations in these websites connect eating with weakness and lack of control, and, therefore, with gaining weight or, by contrast, uncontrolled loss of weight. A study of the advices and instructions on these websites revealed disturbing statistics: 82 % of the websites give a list of "disbeliefs" on which a normal person relies; 47 % offered dangerous solutions; 90 % offered ways to lead parents on; 15 % offered ways to conceal from caregivers [11].

Some of the Pro-Ana websites contain **disclaimer**. It is a warning on the first page, alerting viewers to enter the site at their own risk and informing of the nature of the information on the site. The disclaimer also notes that they should not enter the site if they are recovering from an eating disorder [10]. Norris et al. [8] found that only 58 % of the web pages posted a disclaimer. The seven websites that did post a disclaimer noted that the website supported the Pro-Ana movement, discouraged individuals who had recovered from an eating disorder from entering, and prohibited individuals under age 18 from entering without parental consent.

Several researchers [8, 10, 21, 25] have investigated the content of these websites to determine exactly what kind of messages they are sending and what information they are providing. Mulveen and Hepworth [21] identified several main themes when studying a Pro-Anorexia forum. At the onset of their study there were 15,159 messages posted on the Pro-Anorexia forum and 1,060 registered users. They collected data from 15 separate message threads, which is an original topic posted to a message board as well as other members' replies, during a 6-week period. The first major theme that they noted was **weight loss**. Dietary restriction and special fasts were primary weight loss methods discussed on the forum. Calorie counting was an essential component of messages related to food and fasting. Discussions also centered on the use of diet pills, herbal remedies, and caffeine use in order to increase weight loss. Members also shared their weight goals and ideal body appearance with each other.

Social support was another theme seen in the Pro-Ana forum that Mulveen and Hepworth [21] studied. Members of the online community often referred to the emotional support that they experienced by being part of this online forum. Individuals on the website commented that being able to talk about their eating was helpful in that they were unable to discuss these issues outside the website due to the stigma associated with AN. Direct support was also offered on the website. There was support for eating disordered weight loss as well as support for healthy eating and recovery. "Individuals with eating disorders appear to see Pro-Anorexia sites as an exclusive place where they can experience tremendous personal freedom to be themselves and not have to hide their eating disorder from others, such as from friends, colleagues, and professionals in 'real life'" [21, p. 292]. In another study by Dias [10] it was found that a **desire to have a space** in which they can discuss issues **free from judgment** and **decrease feelings of isolation** were common themes in many of the members' narratives. Although support for recovery was offered for those members who reached dangerously low weights or were getting into more extreme eating disordered behaviors, the website did emphasize the need for AN. Perceived positive aspects of fasting were reported and included achieving weight goals and purification. On the website, AN was perceived as a purifying way of life, both physically and spiritually.

In a similarly conducted analysis of Pro-Anorexia websites Norris et al. [8] identified ten main themes of the 12 Pro-Anorexia websites they reviewed which included; **control, success, perfection, isolation, sacrifice, transformation, coping, deceit, solidarity, and revolution**. All of these themes are related to the themes that Mulveen and Hepworth [21] identified in their research. The theme of **control** was evident in that websites suggested that successful weight loss would lead to control over one's body and life. **Success** was related to strength and measured by weight loss. **Sacrifice** was also a recurrent theme. In order to be successful with AN, one would have to forego their relationships and school. Deceit may also be necessary in order to protect their eating disorder. There was also an emphasis on the idea that eating disorders can transform an individual from being fat and ugly to thin and beautiful. The Pro-Ana websites also viewed the AN as a means of coping and offered ways to cope with the eating disorder rather than treat it. Like the website studied by Mulveen and Hepworth [21], there was an emphasis on **support** and a **judgment free** forum.

Support groups in the Pro-Ana community are usually very active. Another study examined posts in a forum over a 3-day period found that **support** was the most significant and recognized element in the on-going correspondence. Support included compliments and reinforcements to lose weight, encouragement during difficult situations and crisis, and sharing personal experiences as a way of dissipating the feeling of isolation and strengthening a feeling of belonging. Since the lifestyle of those with AN has an obvious physical manifestation, community members turn these phrases into targets in the weight losing process: signs such as hair loss and erratic menstrual cycles represent milestones in the process that demand attention in the forum, leading to explanations and answers to the community participants [18].

The language that is frequently used on these Pro-Ana websites differs significantly from the **language** found on pro-recovery websites. Lyons et al. [27] looked at 162 Internet message board entries and 56 home pages either from Pro-Anorexia websites or from entries of recovering anorexics. These entries were analyzed for linguistic markers of emotional, cognitive, and social functioning, as well as temporal focus and anorexia-related psychological concerns. Pro-Anorexia websites contained more **positive emotional words** in both their homepages and their message board entries. Similarly there were less **anxiety related words** on the pro-anorexia websites compared to the websites of those recovering from the illness. Pro-Anorexia websites contained significantly less **cognitive mechanism words,** especially words concerning insight, than did recovering anorexic websites. **Self-referencing** was more seen on the entries of those recovering from AN compared to those Pro-Anorexia. The focus of the **here and now** was more seen on the homepages and the message boards of the Pro-Ana websites than the pro-recovery entries. As expected Pro-Ana websites also contained many more words associated with eating and made fewer references to school and death-related issues than pro-recovery websites. "The word use of Pro-Anorexics indicated a more pronounced hedonic focus on positive emotions and the here and now, reduced level of cognitive processing, and a lower degree of self-preoccupation" (p. 256).

What Roles Do Pro-Ana Community Serve?

With all of the negative publicity and all of the efforts to ban these sites, why do these sites continue to flourish? To answer this question, it is necessary to look at the role that these websites serve for individuals with AN. As Tierney [28] suggests, individuals with AN often retreat from relationships and situations where their anorexic behaviors can be exposed. Pro-Ana websites are a place where these individuals can identify with others and avoid the isolation that is typically associated with AN. The Pro-Ana website becomes a community for these individuals. The Internet is convenient and available for researching and investigating possible support groups, to which a young girl can easily connect at her own household environment [10]. As Norris et al. [8] note, through the use of fashion accessories, often in the form of a red bracelet, individuals become part of a community that endorses and practices anorexic behaviors. Not only do Pro-Ana websites provide a safe place for individuals with AN to be themselves, but advocates of Pro-Ana sites also claim that the websites minimize risks. As one member describes "giving anorexics a place to go, a place to find support and learn about the disorder….this way hopefully everyone will know how to do this as healthy as possible" [25, p. 963].

There also may actually be a therapeutic component within these websites. In the treatment process its common to have several stages that evoke readiness for change. In the case of AN, in the beginning of treatment the patients are at many times not ready and not willing to participate. During the first stages of the illness these patients usually deny the existence of any problem. They seek support but are unwilling to receive it from the conventional therapy. Generally this results in individuals not getting support unless they are forced into treatment or until they speak to a professional. With Pro-Ana websites, individuals with AN can access less intimidating support before they are ready to seek face-to-face support. Pro-Ana community describes itself as a support group and so the websites are a refuge for those teenage girls that are crying out for help. Pro-Ana websites also frequently discuss AN as 'Ana', a friend, or even a god.

Discussing AN as a separate voice is common on Pro-Ana websites and is also a practice common in Narrative Therapy. In Narrative Therapy patients are encouraged to separate the voice that encourages the destructive behavior, associated with AN from themselves in order to gain some psychological distance and recognize that the eating disorder does not define who they are. Although the public has fought to ban these sites from search engines, very little research has focused on why they exist and what function they serve. As evidenced by the sites themselves, individuals feel that these websites provide them with a space to meet free from judgment where they can support each other and decrease the isolation that they feel [10].

Where Do We Go from Here?

The Internet is a legitimate meeting place, as well as an arena for corporation. Different groups unify around a common subject and discuss it through diverse tools [29]. The power of the virtual community is its ability to contribute to every member in different way, emotionally, cognitively and behaviorally. Nevertheless, when the community's purpose is not socially acceptable, the advantages of the community become controversial. Such is the Pro-Ana community that provides emotional support such as information on losing weight, as well as an encouragement to do so, and sees AN as a legitimate lifestyle.

As Norris et al. [8] indicate many of these websites offer and promote a community of support for anorexics, which allow the perpetuation of the illness in the absence of treatment. Although the websites do provide support, they also allow information to be posted that has the potential to cause short-term and long-term medical complications. Only 58 % of the Pro-Ana websites even had disclaimers about the nature of the website, which is cause for concern given the impact that this type of information can have. Martijn et al. [22] examined the effect of the warning text before visiting Pro-Ana websites on actual access of these websites. A separate webpage with a warning placed before each Pro-Anorexia website hosted by specific provider for a period of 1 year. Of the total number of hits registered at the warning webpage, about one-third of the visitors did not continue to a Pro-Anorexia website. It seems that placement of a warning text before Pro-Anorexia websites can be one of the strategies in holding back visitors.

The nature of the content and the easy accessibility of these websites are worrying. A study that conducted a content analysis of the 'Tips & Tricks' section of Pro-Anorexia websites showed that this information is important for clinicians. Awareness to this information might better equip clinicians to recognize the symptoms of AN early in treatment. Knowledge of 'Tips & Tricks' can also facilitate grater education, making it difficult for clients to conceal their illness [30].

The use of Pro-Anorexia websites by individuals with AN reinforces their existing eating-disordered identity and makes it difficult to change. Tierney [28] emphasizes that clinicians working with AN patients have to convince those who do not necessarily want help that change is possible and is in fact desirable. He also suggests that clinicians working with eating disordered patients should always ask their patients about their use of online resources to see whether they are accessing Pro-Ana websites.

Based on the research field, Pro-Ana web-sites serve an important function for those who suffer from eating disorders. History has shown that these Pro-Ana sites cannot be completely eliminated; therefore, the goal should be to utilize the positive and minimize the negative aspects of these websites. It is important to deepen knowledge with this Pro-Ana community in addition to helping the girls from this community, who came to therapy, to find support other than Pro-Ana's. The more therapists know in this mater, the more they can help their patients to deal with the obligation and the temptation to return to the Pro-Ana community.

Take home points

- The Internet is a legitimate meeting place, as well as an arena for cooperation. Different groups unify around a common subject and discuss it with diverse tools. The power of the virtual community lies in its ability to contribute to every member in different way, emotionally, cognitively and/or behaviorally. When the community's purpose is not socially acceptable, the advantages of the community become controversial.
- Pro-Ana communities provide maladaptive "emotional support" in providing information on losing weight, encouragement to do so, and regarding AN as a legitimate lifestyle.
- Many of these websites offer and promote a community of "support" for individuals with AN, increasing the risk for the perpetuation of the illness in the absence of treatment.
- The nature of the content and the easy accessibility of these websites are worrying.
- The 'Tips & Tricks' section of Pro-Anorexia websites provides important information for clinicians.
- Awareness to this information might better equip clinicians to recognize the symptoms of AN early in treatment.
- Knowledge of 'Tips & Tricks' can also facilitate greater education among clinicans, rendering it difficult for clients to conceal their illness.
- The use of Pro-Anorexia websites by individuals with AN reinforces their existing eating-disordered identity, reducing the likelihood for change.
- Clinicians working with EDs patients should always ask their patients about their use of online resources to find out about the use of Pro-Ana websites.
- Pro-Ana web-sites cannot be completely eliminated; therefore, the goal should be to utilize the positive and minimize the negative aspects of these websites.
- It is important for clinicians to deepen their knowledge about Pro-Ana communies. The more therapists know, the more they can help their patients to deal with the temptation and urge to be linked to Pro-Ana communities.

References

1. Hsu LKG. Eating disorders. New York: Gilford Press; 1990.
2. Hesse-Biber SN, Leavy P, Quinn CE, Zoino J. The mass marketing of disordered eating and eating disorders: The social psychology of women, thinness and culture. Women's Studies International Forum. 2006;29:208–24.
3. Hesse-Biber SN. The cult of thinness. New York: Oxford University Press; 2007.
4. Latzer Y. Eating disorders. Jerusalem: Sold Institute; 1999. (Hebrew).
5. Agras WS. The consequences and costs of the eating disorders. Psychiatr Clin North Am. 2001;24:371–9.
6. Harrison K. Television viewing, fat stereotyping, body shape standards, and eating disorder symptomatology in grade school children. Communication Research. 2000;27:617–40.

7. Holmstrom AJ. The effect of the media on body image: a meta-analysis. Journal of Broadcasting and Electronic Media. 2004;48:196–218.
8. Norris ML, Boydell KM, Pinhas L, Katzman DK. Ana and the Internet: a review of pro-anorexia websites. Int J Eat Disord. 2006;39:443–7.
9. Fox S. Health Information Online.PEW Internet & American Life Project 2005. Accessed July 9, 2008, from http://www.pewinternet.org/pdfs/PIP_Healthtopics_May05.pdf.
10. Dias K. The ana sanctuary: Women's pro-anorexia narratives in cyberspace. Journal of International Women's Studies. 2003;4:31–45.
11. Abbate Daġa G, Gramaglia C, Piero A, Fassino S. Eating disorders and the Internet: Cure and curse. Eating & Weight Disorders, 2006; 11:68–71.
12. Brotsky SR, Giles D. Inside the "Pro-Ana" community: A covert online participant observation. Eating Disorders. 2007;15:93–109.
13. Barak A. Youth and Internet: The psychology of the 'as if' [KE'ILU] and the 'suchlike' [KAZE]. Panim, 2006; 37:48–58. (Hebrew).
14. Steinberg L. Adolescence. Boston: McGraw-Hill; 2008.
15. Valkenburg PM, Peter J. Preadolescents' and adolescents' online communication and their closeness to friends. Dev Psychol. 2007;43:267–77.
16. Bargh JA, McKenna KYA. The Internet and social life. Annu Rev Psychol. 2004;55:573–90.
17. Suler J. The psychology of text relashionships. In: Kraus R, Zack J, Stricker G, editors. Online counseling: A handbook for mental health professionals. San Diego, CA: Elsevier Academic Press; 2004. p. 19–50.
18. Gavin J, Rodham K, Poyer H. The presentation of "pro-anorexia" in online group interactions. Qual Health Res. 2008;18:325–33.
19. Chesley EB, Alberts JD, Klein JD, Kreipe RE. Pro or con? Anorexia Nervosa and the Internet. J Adolesc Health. 2003;32:123–4.
20. Russel J. Treating Anorexia nervosa. British Medical Journal (editorial article). 1995;311:584.
21. Mulveen R, Hepworth J. An interpretative phenomenological analysis of participation in a pro-anorexia Internet site and its relationship with disordered eating. Journal of Health Psychology. 2006;11:283–96.
22. Martijn C, Smeets E, Jansen A, Hoeymans N, Schoemaker C. Don't get the message: the effect of a warning text before visiting a proanorexia website. International Journal of Eating Disorder. 2009;42:139–45.
23. Shirky C. Here comes everybody: the power of organizing without organizations. New-York: The Penguin Press; 2008. p. 202–8.
24. Giles D. Constructing identities in cyberspace: the case of eating disorders. Br J Soc Psychol. 2006;45:463–77.
25. Fox N, Ward K, O'Rourke A. Pro-anorexia, weight loss drugs and the Internet: an 'anti-recovery' explanatory model of anorexia. Sociol Health Illn. 2005;27:944–71.
26. Bardone-Cone AM, Cass KM. Investigating the impact of pro-anorexia websites a pilot study. European Eating Disorders Review. 2006;14:256–62.
27. Lyons EJ, Mehl MR, Pennebaker JW. Pro-anorexia and recovering anorexics differ in their linguistic Internet self-presentation. J Psychosom Res. 2006;60:253–6.
28. Tierney S. The dangers and draw of online communication: Pro-anorexia websites and their implications for users, practitioners, and researchers. Eating Disorders. 2006;14:181–90.
29. Rheingold H. Smart Mobs: the next social revolution. Cambridge: Perseus Publishing; 2002.
30. Harshbarger JL, Ahlers-Schmidt CR, Mayans L, Mayans D, Hawkins JH. Pro-Anorexia websites: What a clinician should know. International Journal on Eating Disorders. 2009;42:367–70.

Chapter 12
Spiritual Self Starvation En-Route to Salvation

Eliezer Witztum, Daniel Stein, Yael Latzer and Moshe Kalian

Abstract The chapter describes the historical background of the relationships between eating disorders and religious and symbolic idioms. Subsequently, the phenomenon termed "spiritual self-starvation" and its linkage to asceticism is described in the context of religious beliefs and practices. The religious aspects of this phenomenon are further elaborated via three cases demonstrating the so-called "Jerusalem Syndrome." Accordingly, their extraordinary visit to Jerusalem has led them to induced fasting and voluntary refusal to eat in the context of sacredness, purification, and penance. The afflicted individuals perceive their distress in terms that construct a narrative integrating self-starvation into their religious and spiritual life. "Spiritual self-starvation" in these cases exceeds the boundaries of religious

E. Witztum (✉)
Division of Psychiatry, Faculty of Health Sciences, Ben Gurion University of the Negev, Beersheba, Israel
e-mail: elyiit@actcom.co.il

E. Witztum
Mental Health Center, Beersheba, Israel

D. Stein
Pediatric Psychosomatic Department, Edmond and Lily Safra Children's Hospital, Chaim Sheba Medical Center, Tel HaShomer, Israel
e-mail: daniel.stein@gmail.com

D. Stein
Sackler Faculty of Medicine, Tel Aviv University, Tel Aviv, Israel

Y. Latzer
Faculty of Social Welfare and Health Sciences, Haifa University, Haifa, Israel
e-mail: latzery@gmail.com

Y. Latzer
Institute for the Treatment and Study of Eating Disorders, Division of Psychiatry, Rambam Health Care Campus, Haifa, Israel

M. Kalian
Israel Society of Forensic Psychiatry, Jerusalem, Israel

Y. Latzer and D. Stein (eds.), *Bio-Psycho-Social Contributions to Understanding Eating Disorders*, DOI 10.1007/978-3-319-32742-6_12

devoutness to the extent of self-endangering psychotic attitudes and behaviors. The significance of Jerusalem as a unique sacred space where according to religious eschatology, great events are about to occur, may lead premorbidly vulnerable individuals to enactments that are reflected in their utilization of the holy space for personal salvation as well as for global redemption.

Introduction

Historical Survey

A historical survey of eating disorders reveals that symptoms and syndromes of self-starvation are not a recent phenomenon. In the following section, we will describe significant landmarks in the history of self-starvation, with a specific emphasis on the motivations for self-starvation in different eras [26].

Self-starvation was virtually unknown in the classical world. Some cases of post-eating vomiting were described in the Roman period, but no reminiscent of anorexia nervosa (AN) are mentioned. Extreme behaviors related to fasting and self-starvation emerged only when European cultures begun to be influenced by Eastern religions. These religions preached a dichotomy between the material world as perceived by the senses, and the eternal, sacred reality of the soul, trapped in the human body. The Gnostic sects, who became particularly popular following the Roman conquest of Greece, advocated that wisdom and knowledge (gnosis) leading to true salvation are entrapped in a world that was basically evil and corrupt. The Gnostic belief in the dichotomy between the evil, corrupt material world and the inner spiritual entity had a tremendous effect on the early Christians, who preferred to withdraw from the sinful city life to remote, secluded sites.

The practice of self-starvation as a means for purification and spiritual seeking is found in biographies of the first Christian monks, such as Hilarion and his contemporaries. Under Christian guise, Gnostic ideas infiltrated the Roman world. For example, St. Jerome (the translator of the Bible from Hebrew into Latin), became in the fourth century AD the spiritual 'guru' for a group of wealthy Roman ladies. Records describe a young Roman girl of an upper-class family who fasted to her death as a result of the implementation of St. Jerom's extreme ascetic doctrine—perhaps the first documented description of willful self-starvation. The girl's death enforced Jerome to flee from Rome to Bethlehem [5].

Self-starvation as a Religious Idiom

Asceticism may be defined as a doctrine in which a person can attain a high spiritual and moral state by practicing self-denial and self-mortification. It implies a spiritual foundation for the practices it denotes, but the precise nature of the foundation of asceticism is obscure. It is certain that its origins antedate and extend beyond the confines of Judeao-Christian tradition, although it is within the context of the Catholic faith that ascetic practices have influenced the moral values of western civilization, through their demonstration in the lives of saints and other venerated persons [19].

The Gnostic-Christian attitude of despising the human flesh as a source of evil and as an obstacle for redemption marked European cultures for hundreds of years, and is still significant in the contemporary secular world. Indeed, different forms of anorectic behaviors became common towards the end of the Middle-Ages and during the Renaissance. A considerable number of the women involved in these behaviors were canonized as saints, and their biographies were circulated by their priest-confessors as a model to others. A famous case was that of St. Catherine of Sienna. Born in 1397 as the twenty-fourth daughter of a prosperous merchant family, she began fasting at the age of 16 years, subsequent to two tragic events that occurred in rapid succession—the death of a beloved older sister in childbirth, and the death of a younger sister. Shortly after these heartbreaking events, Catherine, who came of age by the standards of her time, was destined by her parents to get married. She strongly opposed their decision, (an act sharply disapproved by her family), and then started fasting, spending long hours in devout praying as well as punishing her body with flagellation and other forms of self-abuse. Eventually her parents gave their permission that she would become a nun. However, she died of malnutrition at the age of 32. Her internal experiences of self-starvation were well-documented, since she was a prolific and abled writer. Catherine refused to eat because she considered herself afflicted by an inability to eat. Instead, she devoted herself to caring for the sick, the poor, and the miserable, in complete self-negation and disregard for her own needs. Her need for absolute self-control can clearly be seen in some of the stories about her, as well as the total suppression of her bodily urges [3].

In later years, there were cases of other women refusing eating due to "divine" reasons that were declared as saints. According to Bell and Bynum, peers and superiors of the fasting saints attempted repeatedly to convince these women to eat, sometimes even by force, to avoid the sin of vainglory, an inability to engage in holy responsibilities, or the sin of suicide.

These cases show that religious themes and symbolisms may be very significant in the construction of this type of willful self-starvation. As such, it is not surprising that religious themes and symbolisms are currently often still observed among individuals diagnosed with eating disorders [10] whereas in some of these individuals there is a genuine association between religious beliefs and self-starvation, others may utilize religious concepts consciously to account for their eccentric behavior. Moreover, in some specific groups, restrictions of food intake may be particularly holy, pure and blessed. Still, people involved in acts of fasting may vary in their religious and cultural backgrounds, as well as in the extent to which their families regard the importance of religiosity [2]. In some cases, religious beliefs seem to provide containment of maladaptive behaviors such as fasting through prayers and religious rituals. In such cases, it proves difficult to separate the concepts of a punitive God and bizarre religious explanatory models from the illness process per se. Extreme cases of self-starvation using religious explanatory models can be regarded as forms of "spiritual starvation" [17].

Food is a fundamental concern in many religions. In Christianity, food practice —fasting and feasting—was at the very heart of Christian tradition. According to Bell [3] and Bynum [6] there was a connection between religious asceticism and voluntary starvation by women in Western Europe during the medieval and early modern periods. Bynum describes that during the 13th and 14th centuries, a good Christian was expected to fast on certain days and receive communion at least once a year. Food was a central metaphor and symbol in Christian poetry, devotional literature and theology because a meal (the Eucharist or Lord's Super as a symbol of Christ's body and blood) was a central Christian ritual—the most direct way of encountering the Lord [6].

Bell observes that the majority of women canonized as saints by the Roman Catholic Church in Italy between the 13th century and the present had anorectic behavior patterns. He labels the type of self-starvation and refusal to eat typified by those women as "holy anorexia", and claims that the rationale for self-starvation and fasting was grounded in religious precepts and practices, especially in the literature of radical ascetic Christian religiosity. In her study of the food-related religious practices of European women during the same period, Bynum locates the food asceticism of women in the sexual division of labor and proposes that food was important to women religiously because it was important socially [1].

Clinicians emphasize that asceticism may reach extreme forms in people with AN [7, 18–20]. Palazzoli comments on the ascetic element of AN that reflects a rigid belief in a split between the body and mind. This dualistic logic leads the individual with AN to believe that "one has only to crush the one (the strong body) to enhance the other (the weak spirit), thus magically reversing their respective roles" [18]. Sabom notes the tendency of people with AN to bifurcate the mind and spirit from the body, and to reject the body [20]. Bemporad and Ratey [4] describe in people with AN the sense of moral superiority derived from the endurance of painful abnegation and the relinquishment of gratification of desires; self-control is praised, while any form of indulgence is disapproved. Mogul, proposes that AN may be an extreme form of asceticism that becomes an end in itself [16]. Indeed, people with AN may understand and express their self-starvation in religious terms and construct it as a part of a spiritual messianic mission for redemption. From a different perspective, such spiritual messianic self-starvation may be observed also in extreme forms of the so-called Jerusalem Syndrome.

Jerusalem Syndrome

The so-called "Jerusalem syndrome" is a rather dramatic, cultural–religious phenomenon, rarely appearing in pilgrims and tourists visiting this Holy City in Israel.

Jerusalem serves as the arena in which pre-germinated messianic ideations may be acted out [23–25]. Messianic aspirations in which the Holy City, Jerusalem, the "axis mundi" of faith, is perceived as the arena where great dramatic events are about to occur, are Integral within the Judeo-Christian tradition [13]. This eschatological core element is at times exploited in a broader sense in the service of a public or an individual, to the extent where boundaries between reality and imagination may be blurred [23, 24]. For some vulnerable individuals (mostly with previous psychiatric history), the extraordinary and overwhelming mental experience of facing the holy space of Jerusalem may yield an emotional response exceeding the fragile individual's ability to adequately cope with it. This reaction is often characterized by identification with significant biblical or messianic figures and can yield fantastic behaviors [26]. Earlier descriptions of the so-called Jerusalem Syndrome go back as far as the Middle Ages [13] with an increase in its appearance noted since the revival of the Holy Land tourism during the 19th century [23, 24].

Many descriptions of the Jerusalem Syndrome encompass elements of religion-related self-starvation. Perhaps the earliest detailed "case" of the syndrome is that of Ranieri, the patron of Pisa, who displayed an admixture of piety and unusual behaviour while in Jerusalem in the 12th century and lived for 20 years on stale bread and water. The first medical descriptions of the syndrome are recorded by Dr Heinz Herman, a pioneer psychiatrist in the land of Israel during the early decades of the 20th century [14]. In modern research, it has been noted that about 18 % of the tourists who need psychiatric hospitalization in Jerusalem display significant features of the syndrome, in severe cases, involuntary hospitalization is required [12]. In the next section we present three descriptions of people displaying the Jerusalem Syndrome involving beliefs and behaviors associated with self-starvation [14].

"Mary"—"To Die of Famine on the Streets of Jerusalem" [14]

A foreign woman in her mid-sixties was found on a cold winter day lying on a street bench in Jerusalem, thin, pale, and obviously suffering from the cold weather. She was mute and refusing to answer questions; eventually she was brought by the authorities to a general hospital. There, she was treated for two weeks for hypothermia and malnutrition. Once stabilized, she began to speak in English only of her religious ideation that God had intended for her "to die of famine on the streets of Jerusalem", which she had attempted to do. She expressed puzzlement at the fact that she had been rescued from death, understanding this as another message from God, but one with unclear meaning to her. She was transferred to a mental health facility while attempts were made to contact her family abroad. When examined, she was preoccupied with the belief of being chosen to do difficult things by God, her relationship with God, and God's plans for her life. However, she vehemently denied ever hearing commanding voices, and described "an inner feeling" of what she was supposed to do. Her affect was somewhat labile, jumping from tears at tragic events, to ecstasy when speaking of her religious revelations, to feeling confused when asked about why she thought she was hospitalized when God had truly intended for her to die. She admitted mood swings and that there were times when she would become "extremely happy". Her speech was fast, expansive, and highly gestured, and she often showed a flight of ideas. Virtually every sentence was peppered with biblical analogy, proverb, or grammar and syntax intended to approximate King James English, though she often mixed up biblical stories. Any attempt to ask her a practical question would be answered in a way that would return to a religious statement or theme. There were some idiosyncratic uses of language and phrasings reflecting possible disordered thinking. She had an accent consistent with the highly educated classes of her native country, which was comically incongruous when coupled with the fundamentalist religious content of her thoughts and speech. After a few days of treatment, she was able to give a clear life history, although relating everything and every answer to its religious significance as currently viewed by her. She had no history of any psychological or psychiatric treatment, and no significant medical history, and was generally against modern medicine, believing that whether one lived or died was "in the Lord's hands".

Being brought up in an upper middle-class yet dysfunctional family, she discovered a deep interest in religion at the age of 12, and began to admire rites and rituals of the Catholic Church, strongly wishing to convert, against the will of her non-practicing Episcopalian parents. Her father stated that "religion is for the weak", yet finally her parents gave in and let her convert to Catholicism in her teens. She entered a prestigious university after high school, and studied for two years (accounting for her accent), and then left to get married. She had two children, when she became interested for a year or two in a fundamentalist Christian sect, converting again, only to lose interest shortly after. She tied her religious revelation and the start of the development of her own religious views to an experience she had on a specific date in the 1970s. She described standing in her kitchen and suddenly receiving an overwhelming feeling of divine love, and abundance, and knowing that she had been chosen for a special destiny. She knew that she was to be the bride of Christ, and became increasingly involved with her own religious ideas. After her children were grown, she and her husband divorced. She claimed that "He had free will, and he had to leave, because the Lord was not first in his life, and he could not love the Lord more than he loved me, and I could not stay with him like that".

After several years of self-imposed isolation in the large former family home, she decided that it was her destiny to go to Jerusalem. She described the period leading up to that revelation as the time when she realized that she was meant to cut away from people to be closer to Him. "My sin was loving my children more than Him. Peculiar people set aside in the wilderness to carry a cross. It is so lonely when you have to carry the burden of the Lord. I was proud, I rebelled. I learned at that time not to". At some point, without notifying anyone, she boarded a plane to Israel. She wandered the streets of Jerusalem for 6 years. She stayed for a time with an elderly woman who apparently liked her company and tolerated her religious eccentricities, until 1 day, "God told me I was getting too close to her, so I left while she was sleeping and never came back". She became increasingly isolated, and simultaneously increasingly involved in her relationship with God.

Eventually, in the middle of winter, she came to believe that she "was meant to die of famine on the streets of Jerusalem". When famine was not quick enough in coming, she knew that she was supposed to starve herself and die for God. She did not claim to understand the command or to have a theological underpinning of it, but just knew that this was her destiny, and that sentence—"to die of famine on the streets of Jerusalem"—obsessed her. She decided to sit down on a sheltered bench and wait for death to come, and had been doing so for an undetermined amount of time until she finally hospitalized. When questioned about her motives, she denied direct suicidal ideation, and said that "Love for other people is the sword that divides. One must love only the Lord, like David who loved his family and had to be separated, to be delivered from one's wretched flesh. Dying is salvation from the body. Death is our next stage, we become better creatures".

During her hospitalization, her country's embassy was contacted, and it was discovered that her children had filed a missing person report on her at the time of her original disappearance. They had not suspected foul play, but rather that she was most likely living with a religious cult of one sort or another. They were contacted, and one family member agreed to come to Israel to bring her home. When asked about her future plans, she seemed confused, yet hopeful that she could be reunited with her family "like Joseph and his brothers. God knows how much I want to be with them. I've never hung on to my family and my parents never hung on to me. Like David running away to God because God is more merciful than man. But I don't understand, why was I supposed to come here but now I am being sent back there? I just don't fit anywhere". About the wisdom of her starvation attempt, she said, "I tend to jump into things, and He's always telling me to work on that. But mercy triumphs over justice". A relative arrived in Israel, revealing that her house was still in her possession, having stood empty for these six years. He dealt with the bureaucracy of obtaining a replacement passport for her, and returned with her to their country [14].

"Abraham Son of Abraham"—"To Regain One's Jewish Soul" [14]

Right after being located by the police, "Abraham son of Abraham" was taken to a general hospital due to severe dehydration and extreme self-neglect. It turned out that for several days, he was spotted by visitors and local residents in the Old City of Jerusalem, who reported his condition to the police. Though accustomed to eccentric figures occasionally wandering in the local neighborhood, Abraham's condition raised concern. He was a big man, seemed to be in his fifties, and would sit motionless for hours in the street, seldom changing place or positions. No one knew where he came from. He did not respond to people approaching him, his eyes were closed, and he seemed to murmur words to himself. No one saw him eat or drink. He was a huge man in a state of extreme physical neglect, with a total lack of hygiene, unwashed and malodorous, with filthy clothes, long greasy grey hair and a long unclean beard. He did not respond to people talking to him and kept his eyes shut. Yet, when finally approached by the police, he did not resist being held by them and sent to the emergency room. After a general checkup and fluid infusion, it became clear that his problem was mainly a mental one, and he was referred to a psychiatric ward. He was diagnosed as being in a catatonic state and was treated accordingly. Within a few days of treatment, he became more cooperative, began to eat and drink, and responded verbally in English. His behavior became more expressive and flamboyant, at times standing up with his arms raised towards the ceiling and his eyes wide open as he was talking to God. Though still suspicious and rather withdrawn, some rapport was possible. During the interviews, he became very selective with the information he had given, claiming that any detailed answers regarding his past would harm his family. According to his version, he was a Protestant by birth, suffering from schizoaffective disorder diagnosed in his youth. He was first hospitalized shortly after graduating from law school. He believed the trigger at that time was a romantic disappointment. Since then, there were several recurrent schizoaffective episodes and hospitalizations.

For years, he searched for one true love. In his seeking, he gradually approached Judaism, believing he had found a path to the true love of God. His first visit to the Holy Land was 4 years ago, when he joined a certain religious sect in Jerusalem. However, he was forced to return to his country once his means ran out. According to his story, about a year prior to his current visit to Jerusalem, he converted to Judaism. Yet, being forced to return home, he became alarmed by the thought that his own Jewish soul had been stolen and found its way into another gentile's body. He felt that he must return to Holy Jerusalem, where he should fast and praise the Lord until his body becomes pure enough to regain the Jewish soul stolen from him. While fasting and praying in the streets of the Holy City, he was elated by the experience that cherubim mingled all around him. He was not aware of his physical condition, yet believed that it was the hand of the Lord that interfered in the last moment, saving his deteriorated yet purified body to regain his soul. For a while, after confiding his story and expressing his wish to live in Jerusalem, Abraham perceived the local hospital staff as his allies. However, once it became clear that in spite of all his efforts, the Israeli authorities wanted him to be sent back to his native country (this because his conversion to Judaism was questionable, he had no means to support himself, and his visa had expired), Abraham's attitude changed greatly. He began to perceive the staff as hostile, "plotting" and persecutory, and could not forgive their "betrayal". He then became very aggressive towards the staff and other "hostile" patients and had to be transferred to a maximum-security ward, located outside Jerusalem, before being sent back to his country [14].

"The Repenting Ebenezer—To Reach Jerusalem in Heaven"

Ebenezer was a good-looking young and athletic university student, who was brought to the emergency room in a general hospital in Jerusalem by his neighbors at the dormitory. It turned out that for several days, he did not step out of him room, gave up going to lectures and other duties, stopped eating and was indulged in fasting and praying. When found by his peers, he was already quite weak and mildly dehydrated. His hospitalization was only a short time after he came to Jerusalem from West-Africa in a student exchange program.

Ebenezer was the eldest son and a third generation of an African middle-class family converted to Methodist Christianity. His parents were devoutly religious, highly educated and with western orientation, and transmitted high expectations from their children. Ebenezer was a very good student at school and it was only natural that he would be accepted to a prestigious university faculty. Like his parents he was a devout Christian and became even more devout since adolescence. There was an inner feeling in him that he was destined by God to help the poor, the ill and the suffering, yet remained humble though highly valued by his family and community.

The young bright student chose to study medicine. Although being considered a brilliant student in pre-academic days, he found university schooling tremendously difficult, at the verge of failure. Ebenezer began to be fascinated with the life of the Savior, and hoped that in due time he would be able to visit the Holy Land and walk in the footsteps of Jesus. Then "as a sign from God", there came an exciting opportunity to go to Jerusalem in a student exchange program.

The meeting with the Holy City puzzled Ebenezer completely. It was an earthly domain, inhabited by regular people of different cultures and affiliations, carrying regular secular life and domestic routines with no trace or sign of the Glory he anticipated. Furthermore, studying was no less difficult than at home. While praying to God and deliberating, an "illumination" approached his mind, pointing that his arrival to the earthly Jerusalem was just a stage in the mission to reach the true spiritual Jerusalem, the one which is "in the sky". He then secluded himself in his room, praying and fasting, withdrawn from any pleasure of the flesh, to be worthy of the mission set for him by God to bring the redemption.

Discussion

Socio-cultural aspects of AN are traditionally associated with the long-standing discussion of whether it can be regarded as representing a culture-dependent syndrome, namely a syndrome that cannot be understood separated from its cultural context [21], or as an idiom of distress, enabling women to express their distress and deal with its consequences by channeling them into numerous eating-related attitudes and behaviors [26]. However, in this chapter we deal with a different socio-cultural aspect of willful self-starvation and refusal to eat, namely their association with religious beliefs and practices.

In early literature on AN, links between spirituality and religion were very clear, and the examination of historical figures led to retrospective diagnoses of AN in some Catholic saints [3, 15, 19]. Rampling had even theorized about the religious context of the relationship between asceticism and AN [19].

We assume that the religious experience and its practices in the three cases described in this chapter may serve as an idiom of distress in their psychotic process, giving sacred meanings to their self-starvation. These individuals connect religious experiences to their highly personal reality, thus offering themselves means of coping with their disorder or at the very least confronting it, on both existential and practical levels. The afflicted individuals have perceived their disorder in terms that may construct a narrative integrating the "experience" into their religious lives [23, 24]. These patients can integrate the disorder into their spiritual life in such a way that they do not have to look at themselves as being insane. In effect, the use of a religious idiom of distress to account for their adaptive behavior, enables them to remain within the framework of the world in which they feel a part in spite of the disruptions resulting from their disorder [9].

A form of idiosyncratic beliefs or delusions can be attributed to issues of food consumption and religiosity. Van Deth and Vandereycken [22] discuss the occurrence of food refusal ("Sitophobia") in Victorian asylums. They claim that food refusal in these instances has been often related to religious ideation, such as fasting and penance for sins committed in the past.

Food refusal can be related not only to eating disorders but also to melancholic or psychotic disorders. William James called asceticism "a symptom of saintliness." [11]. He claimed that in moderate degrees, it is natural and even usual for the human nature to support ascetic attitudes and practices: "asceticism symbolizes the belief that there is an element of real wrongness in this world" that should be corrected. it can be constructed as "a way of living based upon voluntary abstention from sensual, physical pleasures and emphasizing simplicity and self-discipline". The ascetic usually professes to be focusing on a higher moral/religious value system [10].

The narratives of the three cases demonstrate a form of psychotic asceticism leading to self-starvation. Their narratives are idiosyncratic and private, give them a special role in contrast to others, and are out of step with current religious thinking [8]. Their "spiritual self-starvation" exceeds boundaries of religious devoutness to the extent of psychotic self-endangering behaviors The significance of the Holy City of Jerusalem as the arena for extraordinary enactments is reflected in their employment of the holy space, either for global redemption (as in "Mary's case) or for private salvation (as in the case of "Abraham son of Abraham" and "The repenting Ebenezer"). During the psychotic phase, performing self-starvation upon the stage "where great events are about to occur" has become is a powerful element in their spiritual existence. The intervention of local medical and psychiatric agencies, while saving their lives, may leave these individuals in a perplexed world, facing what is apparently an irresolvable conflict.

Take Home Points

- Self-starvation and refusal to eat related to socio-cultural aspect associated with religious believes and practices.
- Early literature on AN links between spirituality, religion, asceticism and self-starvation.
- We suggest that religious experience and practices may serve as an idiom of distress, giving sacred meaning to self-starvation.
- The use of religious idiom of distress to account for an adaptive behavior may enable AN patient to remain within the framework of the world.
- Idiosyncrasies beliefs can be attributed to issues of food consumption and religiosity.

References

1. Banks CG. "There is no fat in heaven": religious asceticism and the meaning of anorexia nervosa. Ethos. 1996;24(1):107–35.
2. Baxter H. Religion and eating Disorder. Eur Eat Disord Rev. 2001;9:137–9.
3. Bell RM. Holy anorexia. Chicago: University of Chicago Press; 1985.
4. Bemporad J, Jules R. Intensive psychotherapy of former anorexic Individuals. Am J Psychother. 1985;39(4):454–66.
5. Bemporad JR. Cultural and historical aspects of eating disorders. Theor Med. 1997;18:401–20.
6. Bynum C. Holy feast and holy fast. The religious significance of food to medieval women. Berkeley, Los Angeles, London: University of California Press; 1987.
7. Garner DM. Eating disorders inventory-2 (EDI-2). Odessa, FL: Psychological Assessment Resources; 1991.
8. Greenberg D, Witztum E. Sanity and Sanctity: Mental health care of the ultra-orthodox community in Jerusalem. New Haven: Yale University Press; 2001. p. 37–51.
9. Heilman S, Witztum E. All in faith: Religion as the idiom and means of coping with distress. Mental Health, Relig Cult. 2000;3:115–24.
10. Huline-Dickens S. Anorexia nervosa: Some connections with the religious attitude. Br J Med Psychol. 2000;73:67–76.
11. James W. The varieties of religious experience. New York: Longman; 1902.
12. Kalian M, Witztum E. Facing a holy space: psychiatric hospitalization of tourists in Jerusalem. In: Kedar BZ, Werblowsky RJZ, editors. Sacred space: Shrine, city, land. Jerusalem & London: Israel Academy of Science and Humanities and Macmillan: 1998. pp. 316–30.
13. Kalian M, Witztum E. Jerusalem Syndrome as reflected in the pilgrimage and biographies of four extraordinary women from the 14th century to the end of the second millennium. Mental Health, Relig Cult. 2002;5:1–16.
14. Kalian M, Catinari S, Heresco-Levi U, Witztum E. Spiritual Starvation" in a Holy Space—a Form of "Jerusalem Syndrome. Mental Health, Relig Cult. 2008;11(2):161–72.
15. Lacey JH. Anorexia nervosa and a bearded female saint. Br Med J. 1982;285:1816–7.
16. Mogul SL. Asceticism in adolescence and anorexia nervosa. Psychoanal Study Child. 1980;35:155–75.
17. Morgan JF, Marsden P, Lacey JH. "Spiritual starvation?": A case series concerning Christianity and eating disorders. Int J Eat Disord. 2000;28:476–80.

18. Palazzoli MS. Self-Starvation. From individual to family therapy in the treatment of anorexia nervosa. New York: Jason Aronson, 1978.
19. Rampling D. Ascetic Ideals and Anorexia Nervosa. J. Psychiatr. Res. 1985;19:89–94.
20. Sabom WS. The gnostic world of anorexia nervosa. J Psychol Theol. 1985;13(4):243–54.
21. Swartz L. Anorexia nervosa as a culture-bound syndrome. Soc Sci Med. 1985;20:725–30.
22. Van Deth R, Vandereycken W. Food refusal and insanity: Sitophobia and anorexia nervosa in Victorian asylums. Int J Eat Disord. 2000;27:390–404.
23. Witztum E, Goodman Y. Narrative construction of distress and therapy: a model based on work with ultra-orthodox jews. Transcult Psychiatry. 1999;36:403–36.
24. Witztum E, Kalian M. The "Jerusalem syndrome"—fantasy and reality. A survey of accounts from the 19th century to the end of the Second Millennium. Israel J Psychiatry. 1999;36:260–71.
25. Witztum E, Kalian M. The Quest for redemption: Reality and Fantasy in the Mission to Jerusalem. In: Hare PA, Kressel GM, editors. Israel as center stage. A setting for social and religious enactment. Westport, CT: Bergin and Grav: 2001. pp. 15–29.
26. Witztum E, Latzer Y, Stein D. Anorexia nervosa and bulimia nervosa as idioms of distress: From the historical background to current formulations. Int J Child Adolesc Heath. 2008;1:283, 94.

Chapter 13
Body Dissatisfaction and Disordered Eating Among Jewish Women: The Role of Religious Orientation and Spiritual Well-Being

Sarah L. Weinberger-Litman, Laura A. Rabin, Joshua Fogel and Janell L. Mensinger

Abstract Numerous psychological, cultural, and biological variables have been investigated in the etiology of eating disorders (EDs) and their risk factors such as body dissatisfaction and a preoccupation with weight and appearance. Despite its historical link to EDs, the role of religion has largely been ignored. Most studies investigating religious influences on ED symptoms use the terms religion and spirituality interchangeably and do not include Jewish women. Studies that have included Jewish women used a single variable (e.g., attendance at religious service) to measure religiosity, which does not adequately capture the nature of one's religious beliefs and practices. In a sample of 301 adolescent and young Jewish women, this study assessed participants' religious orientation and spiritual beliefs to elucidate the possible differential influences of these variables on body dissatisfaction and disordered eating. Results revealed that participants with an intrinsic religious orientation had consistently lower scores (indicating less pathology) on

S.L. Weinberger-Litman · L.A. Rabin
Department of Psychology, Brooklyn College and the Graduate Center of the City University of New York, Brooklyn, NY, USA

S.L. Weinberger-Litman (✉)
Department of Psychology, Marymount Manhattan College, 221 E71st Street, New York, NY 10021, USA
e-mail: sarahleahw@gmail.com

J. Fogel
Department of Economics, Brooklyn College of the City University of New York, Brooklyn, NY, USA

J. Fogel
Department of Earth and Environmental Sciences, Graduate Center of the City University of New York, New York, NY, USA

J.L. Mensinger
Department of Medicine, Reading Hospital and Medical Center, Reading, PA, USA

Y. Latzer and D. Stein (eds.), *Bio-Psycho-Social Contributions to Understanding Eating Disorders*, DOI 10.1007/978-3-319-32742-6_13

measures of body dissatisfaction and eating disturbance as compared to those with an extrinsic, pro-religious, or anti-religious orientation. High levels of spiritual well-being were moderately associated with lower levels of body dissatisfaction but showed no association with disordered eating. Overall, these findings suggest that having an intrinsic religious orientation may confer protection from eating and body image disturbance.

Introduction

The incidence of eating disorders (EDs) has increased dramatically in the United States, Europe, and other Western nations in recent decades [1–3]. As a result, numerous psychosocial, cultural, and biological variables have been investigated in an attempt to understand the etiology of EDs and their risk factors such as body dissatisfaction and a preoccupation with weight and appearance [4]. Despite its historical link to EDs, the role of religion as a possible developmental influence has received little scientific investigation.

The earliest documented cases of anorexia were associated with religious devotion, self-denial, and asceticism [1]. For example, throughout medieval Europe, food refusal was common among women and almost ubiquitous among female saints [5]. The ability to survive without any or with very little food was considered miraculous and a testament to the sanctity of these women and their actions [1]. After the medieval period, the phenomenon of surviving on little food for religious purposes remained common but was seen mainly in adolescent girls and younger women. By the 16th century, this phenomenon became known as "anorexia mirabilis"—a miraculous loss of appetite. Not until the mid-1800s was this condition widely recognized as a psychiatric illness [1].

It is clear that some women (within the Judeo-Christian tradition) historically have felt the need to deny themselves food and other physical pleasures in order to ensure spiritual or religious acceptance [6]. Modern research suggests that religion is an important variable to consider in ED development. For example, Joughin et al. [7] observed a direct relationship between symptoms of anorexia and religious devotion and an inverse relationship between symptoms of bulimia and religious devotion. Smith et al. [8] found that patients with anorexia reported feeling closer to God whereas patients with bulimia reported feeling estranged from God and religious practice. The authors concluded that this observation may be a result of those with anorexia feeling successful in controlling their impulses and transcending their physical needs, which is seen as a virtue in most religious traditions. On the other hand, those with bulimia may feel that they have succumbed to temptation through eating binges and therefore have failed in their quest for impulse control. Therefore, religious influences remain important variables to explore in an attempt to elucidate the etiology of EDs and their risk factors.

Jewish Women and Eating Disorders

The association between religious beliefs and ED symptoms may be especially important to examine among Jewish women. Historically, those of the Jewish faith have had a complex and intimate relationship with food. In addition to special foods associated with the Sabbath and other holidays, observant Jews adhere to strict dietary laws that govern virtually every aspect of food preparation and consumption [9]. While Judaism does not officially endorse asceticism or the denial of physical pleasures, abstaining from food and sex is often mandated as in the case of certain fast days, and can lead, especially among adolescents, to ambivalent feelings about physical needs.

Limited empirical as well as anecdotal evidence suggests that the incidence of EDs among Jewish women, and specifically orthodox Jewish women, is higher than in the general population in the United States [10–12].

Only a handful of studies, however, have focused on ED development among Jewish women, and results have been inconclusive with regard to whether Jewish religious beliefs serve as a protective or vulnerability factor. Gluck and Geliebter [13] found that secular Jewish women had higher rates of anorexic symptoms than their orthodox Jewish counterparts, presumably because of reduced media exposure and less emphasis on physical appearance among orthodox women. Latzer et al. [14] found that among modern orthodox high school girls in Israel, greater levels of religiosity were associated with lower levels of eating pathology. These studies suggest that an increased level of religious observance may be protective against the development of ED symptoms; however, they contradict several anecdotal reports of an inflated prevalence among orthodox women [13, 14]. It is noteworthy however, that these studies explored disordered eating rather than full blown eating disorders. Furthermore, as discussed below, existing studies may be limited by the way religious observance is conceptualized and employed methodologically.

Religious Orientation Versus Religious Observance

The inconsistent findings on the relationship between religion and EDs are similar to what is seen in the larger body of work investigating the relationship between religion and various health outcomes. In a comprehensive review article on the health benefits of religious beliefs [15], the only substantiated finding was that greater attendance at church and religious services was related to a decrease in all-cause mortality. This finding remained even after controlling for the possible behavioral factors associated with church going (i.e. individuals who attend church may have better health habits). There was also a marginally significant association between religious practice and blood pressure but this was greater for women than men. Results have been inconsistent in studies exploring the relationship between religion and cardiovascular disease or cancer [15].

A limiting feature of studies exploring EDs as well as those examining religion and general health outcomes, is that they view religion and religious beliefs as one-dimensional, often assigning a single variable (such as attendance at religious services or self-reported religious observance) as the measure of religiosity [15, 16]. In reality, there may be different types of religious attitudes or beliefs that impact health outcomes. Allport and Ross [17] were among the first to call attention to different types of devotion or religious experiences. In their investigation of religious orientation and personal prejudice, they distinguished between extrinsic and intrinsic religiosity, and designed the religious orientation scale to measure these concepts empirically. According to Allport and Ross, extrinsic individuals "use religion…to provide security, solace, sociability, distraction, status, and self-justification." "Intrinsic" individuals, on the other hand, "live their religion," and "having embraced a creed, the individual endeavors to internalize it and follow it fully" [17]. In other words, extrinsically motivated individuals tend to utilize religion for its social rewards while intrinsically motivated individuals rely on religious beliefs to guide important aspects of their lives. While these terms represent opposite poles, individuals usually fall along an intrinsic/extrinsic continuum, and often endorse a combination of intrinsic and extrinsic characteristics.

Employing a paradigm of religious orientation rather than just observance or behavior may yield a deeper understanding of individuals' underlying religious attitudes and beliefs. Particularly among orthodox Jews, who adhere to a variety of strict guidelines relating to food and other key aspects of life, religious orientation may be a more useful construct than self reported religious observance to investigate the association between religion and EDs. In other populations, religious orientation has been used to examine ED development in a handful of studies. Smith et al. [18] found that women characterized as intrinsically religious tended to have less ED pathology than those characterized as extrinsically religious. Additionally, individuals characterized as pro-religious (who endorsed both intrinsic and extrinsic items on the religious orientation scale), had the highest scores on ED and body image questionnaires. This relationship was observed in both clinical and non-clinical samples. Additionally, Forthun et al. [19] found that intrinsic religiosity decreased the likelihood of developing EDs among women considered to have family risk factors for eating disturbances. Not only was an intrinsic orientation protective in this situation, but extrinsic religiosity appeared to exacerbate these risk factors [19].

While these studies raise compelling issues about the nature of religious orientation and EDs, the samples consisted almost exclusively of individuals from Christian denominations. Thus, one of our goals was to extend this paradigm to Jewish women in order to assess the generalizability of this model and to elucidate the complex association between eating behaviors and religious orientation among Jewish women. We also sought to expand the repertoire of research tools available to study religious influences on EDs and general health given the inconsistencies in the existing literature.

Religiosity Versus Spirituality

A second flaw in the general literature on religion and health, which has implications for ED research, is the confounding of the terms religion and spirituality. In the majority of research studies, the independent variable is referred to as "religion/spirituality" as if they were a single entity. Researchers often aggregate religion and spirituality because of the difficulty in operationalizing and measuring each construct separately [16]. Practically speaking, one could argue that spirituality is experienced on a personal level and involves "transcendence" (e.g., of the physical or material world), while religion occurs on more of a social or public level and is associated with practice, religious ritual, or organized religion [16]. To our knowledge, research has not examined the role that spirituality plays in the development of disordered eating. Accurate clarification and measurement of these distinct concepts would be useful both theoretically and methodologically.

Therefore, an important goal of the current study was to distinguish between religious and spiritual beliefs in order to elucidate the possible differential influences of each on body dissatisfaction and disordered eating.

This study has two overall hypotheses. First, we hypothesize that Jewish women with an intrinsic religious orientation will have lower scores on measures of eating and body image disturbance than any other religious orientation group; conversely, those with an extrinsic religious orientation will have the highest scores of any group. Second, spirituality, as distinct from religion, has rarely been explored as a possible influence on ED development. We hypothesize that Jewish women with high levels of spiritual well-being will have lower scores on measures of eating and body image disturbance than those with low levels of spiritual well-being.

Method

Participants

Participants were 301 Jewish women from three educational settings (i.e., two universities and one high school) in the New York City boroughs of Brooklyn and Manhattan. These establishments were included based on their proximity to the principal investigator's institution and/or because the administrators gave approval for the study. Most participants (n = 185, 61.5 % of the total sample) were drawn from a public 4-year co-educational college that is part of a large city university system. A smaller percentage of participants (n = 43, 14.3 % of the total sample) were enrolled at a private, single-gender college that is also part of a larger university system. The remaining participants (n = 73, 24.3 % of the total sample) were students at a single-gender religious high school (i.e., "Yeshiva").

Procedure

Institutional Review Board approval for the study was received from the first author's main institutional affiliation. Data were collected from August 2006 through March 2007 by the principal investigator and several advanced undergraduate research assistants. All participants were informed that the study entailed completing a series of paper-and-pencil questionnaires that would take approximately 30–45 min on the topic of body image and eating disorders. Participation was completely voluntary and confidential, and informed consent was obtained from all participants.

College-Specific Procedures

The public 4-year college participants were introductory psychology students who received class credit or students recruited from various public sites across campus including the cafeteria, library, and café. With the permission of professors in the Psychology and Judaic Studies departments, participants also were recruited from various undergraduate courses. Individuals not receiving course credit were not compensated for their participation. Participants had the option of completing the questionnaires on campus or off site (in which case they would return the in an envelope provided by the investigators). The private college participants were psychology students who completed the questionnaires during class with the permission of professors familiar with the study. All students approached agreed to participate in the study.

High School-Specific Procedures

Several visits were made to the high school during which the principal investigator provided general background information to students and consent forms for parents of students under age 18 years. Students were assured that parental consent forms would be stored separately from questionnaires so that no identifying information would be visible. Potential participants also were informed that decisions about whether or not to participate would have no bearing on academic outcomes. On return visits by the principal investigator, parental consent forms were collected and questionnaires were distributed to students during free class periods, lunch times, and recesses. All students approached agreed to participate in the study.

Measures

Demographic Information

Participants reported their age, height, and weight (which was then used to calculate body mass index (BMI), calculated as kg/m^2), the gender composition of the high school they currently or previously attended (all-girls vs. coed) and amount of television viewed per week (in hours). Self-reported level of religious observance was measured by asking participants to choose from the following categories; Orthodox, Modern Orthodox, Conservative, Reform, Traditional and Non-Affiliated.

Eating Attitudes Test (EAT-26)

The EAT-26 is a widely used measure of disordered eating [20]. The abbreviated EAT-26, which was used in this study, consists of 26 items that form three subscales: Dieting, Bulimia/Food Preoccupation, and Oral Control. Response options include: "always," "usually," "often," "sometimes," "rarely," or "never." Responses are scored from 0 to 3, where answers of "sometimes," "rarely," and "never" = 0, "often" = 1, "usually" = 2, and "always" = 3. Scores range from 0 to 78 for the EAT-26 Total score, from 0 to 39 for the Dieting subscale, from 0 to 18 for the Bulimia subscale, and from 0 to 21 for the Oral Control subscale, with higher scores indicating a greater degree of disordered eating. The EAT has demonstrated high reliability and consistency and is considered an effective screening tool in both clinical and non-clinical populations [20, 21]. In the initial study, Cronbach alpha reliability was 0.90, 0.90, 0.84, and 0.83 for the EAT Total score, and the Dieting, Bulimia, and Oral Control subscales, respectively. Cronbach alpha reliability in this sample was 0.92, 0.86, 0.90, and 0.78 for the EAT Total score and the Dieting, Bulimia, and Oral Control subscales, respectively.

Body Shape Questionnaire (BSQ)

The BSQ is a 34-item scale that measures concerns about body shape and weight. An additional feature is questions specifically related to the experience of feeling fat, which is considered a risk factor for and primary characteristic of eating disorders [22]. Responses are scored on a 6-point Likert type scale with responses ranging from "never = 1" to "always = 6." Total scores on the BSQ range from 34 to 204, with higher scores indicating greater body dissatisfaction. Although exact values are not reported, the BSQ has demonstrated high internal consistency in previous studies [22]. Cronbach alpha reliability in this sample was 0.97.

Religious Orientation Scale (ROS)

The ROS is a 20-item scale that measures intrinsic and extrinsic religiosity and is among the most widely used tests of religious orientation [17]. Individuals considered intrinsic in their orientation are those who "live their religion," while extrinsic individuals are those who "use their religion." The intrinsic subscale consists of nine items and the extrinsic subscale consists of 11 items. In addition to the intrinsic/extrinsic distinction, two additional constructs emerged from the scale after its development and initial use. Unexpectedly, some individuals tended to agree with both intrinsic and extrinsic items and were labeled as indiscriminately pro-religious, whereas other individuals tended to disagree with both types of items and were labeled as anti-religious. Based on these findings, Allport and Ross [17] conceptualized a fourfold typology of religious orientation, which will be used throughout this paper. Cut-off scores on the intrinsic and extrinsic subscales were used to categorize individuals as high or low on each subscale [23]. Individuals scoring high on the Intrinsic subscale and low on the Extrinsic subscale were categorized as intrinsic, individuals scoring high on the Intrinsic and Extrinsic subscales were categorized as pro-religious, individuals scoring low on both subscales were categorized as anti-religious, and individuals scoring high on the Extrinsic and low on the Intrinsic subscale were categorized as extrinsic.

Scores on the ROS range from 20 to 100 for Total score, with lower values indicating a more intrinsic orientation and higher values indicating a more extrinsic orientation. It is important to note that the ROS is a measure of religious orientation or attitude and is not necessarily a reflection of level of observance. The ROS has demonstrated good Cronbach alpha reliability, ranging from 0.69 to 0.93, and has been widely used [23]. In this sample, Cronbach alpha reliability was 0.74, 0.80, and 0.62 for the Total scale, Intrinsic, and Extrinsic subscales, respectively.

Spiritual Well-Being Scale (SWB)

The SWB is a 20-item scale that assesses overall spiritual well-being and also is used as a general quality of life measure [24]. The SWB contains a 10-item subscale for religious well-being (RWB) that assesses well-being in terms of a particular religious affiliation or relationship with God. The second 10-item subscale measures existential well-being (EWB) in terms of an individual's fulfillment or meaning in life, independent of religion. The SWB is scored on a 6 point Likert-type scale with responses ranging from "strongly agree" = 1 to "strongly disagree" = 6. Total SWB scores range from 20 to 120 and from 10 to 60 for the RWB and EWB subscales. For the total SWB and each subscale, cut-off scores are provided for categorizing individuals as low, moderate, or high for each type of spiritual-well-being.

In previous studies, the SWB demonstrated high internal consistency and reliability across samples and has been shown to be an effective measure in various populations and across religious affiliations [24, 25]. In a study by Paloutzian and Ellison [24], Cronbach alpha reliability ranged from 0.89 to 0.94 (total SWB), 0.82 to 0.94 (RWB), and 0.78 to 0.86 (EWB). In this sample, Cronbach alpha reliability was 0.92, 0.92, and 0.86 for the total SWB, RWB, and EWB, respectively.

Beck Depression Inventory (BDI–II)

The BDI-II is one of the most widely used measures of depressive symptoms in both clinical and research settings [26]. While the full BDI-II consists of 21 items, we eliminated one item that related to sexual activity because it was deemed inappropriate for the high school participants. On the BDI-II, respondents choose one of four statements (for each of the items) that best describes their feelings over the past two weeks. Statements are scored from 0 to 3, with higher scores indicating higher levels of depressive symptoms. For the purposes of our study, total scores ranged from 0 to 60. The BDI-II has consistently demonstrated high reliability with Cronbach alpha reported at 0.93 [26]. Cronbach alpha reliability in this sample was 0.91.

State/Trait Anxiety Inventory for Children (STAI-C)

The STAI-C is a widely used measure of both state and trait anxiety. Although the instrument was designed to be used with children and adolescents, the authors agreed that this test was more appropriate for individuals in our sample than the adult version. As well, we decided to use only the trait anxiety scale (T-Anxiety), which measures relatively stable individual differences in anxiety proneness (i.e., differences between individuals in the tendency to experience anxiety states). The T-Anxiety scale consists of 20 items related to emotions and behaviors associated with anxiety. Responses include "hardly-ever" = 1, "sometimes" = 2, and "often" = 3. Total scores range from 20 to 60, with higher scores indicating higher levels of anxiety. While exact alpha values have not been reported, the STAI-C has demonstrated good reliability [27]. In this sample, Cronbach alpha reliability was 0.89.

Statistical Analyses

Analysis of variance (ANOVA) was used to compare group differences in demographic characteristics. We next examined the relationship of eating disorder symptoms to religious orientation and spiritual well-being. Separate ANOVAs were used to evaluate differences for the independent variables of religious orientation and spiritual well-being. Dependent variables were the Eating Attitudes Test (EAT) and the Body Shape Questionnaire (BSQ). When appropriate, Least Significant Difference post hoc tests also were conducted. A second model used analysis of covariance (ANCOVA) and adjusted for the demographic variables of age, BMI, and self-reported religious observance (orthodox Jewish vs. non-orthodox Jewish); data collection site was included as a random effects variable. A third model used ANCOVA and adjusted for the demographic variables in model 2 as well as for depression (as measured by the BDI-II), anxiety (as measured by the STAI-C); data collection site was included as a random effects variable. As appropriate, variables were evaluated for skewness and those that were skewed were logarithmically transformed. SPSS version 15 (SPSS, 2006) was used for all analyses except for calculation of Cohen's d, which used the online Becker Effect Size Calculator [28].

Results

Participant Characteristics

There were no significant differences between participants at any of the data collection sites in terms of body mass index (BMI), $F(2,283) = 0.62$, $p = 0.54$, $\eta^2 = 0.004$, level of eating disturbance, $F(2,298) = 1.03$, $p = 0.36$, $\eta^2 = 0.007$, body image dissatisfaction, $F(2,298) = 0.78$, $p = 0.46$, $\eta^2 = 0.005$, or depressive symptoms, $F(2,298) = 1.19$, $p = 0.31$, $\eta^2 = 0.008$. There was a significant difference for anxiety between the public and private college participants that was controlled for in subsequent analyses, $F(2,298) = 3.13$, $p = 0.05$, $\eta^2 = 0.02$. The mean age of the total sample was 19.00 (SD = 2.42), the means and standard deviations for the Brooklyn College, private college and high school samples were 19.75 (2.00), 20.63 (1.89) and 16.18 (0.94) respectively. The mean body mass index (BMI), measured using self-reported height and weight, was 21.70 (SD = 2.94). The mean depressive symptoms score for the overall sample was 11.32 (SD = 8.86) and the mean anxiety score was 37.25 (SD = 8.13), both of which were below levels suggesting clinical concern. The majority of the sample (76.1 %; n = 229) reported being Orthodox or Modern-Orthodox Jewish, and were categorized as observant, whereas the remainder of the sample endorsed conservative, reform, traditional, non-affiliated, or "other" when questioned about their religious observance and were categorized as non-observant (20.6 %, n = 62).

Religious Orientation and Eating Disorder Symptoms

As shown in Table 13.1, ANOVAs were conducted with religious orientation as the independent variable and each total scale or subscale of the EAT and BSQ as the

Table 13.1 Influence of religious orientation on body dissatisfaction and eating disturbance

	Intrinsic M (SD)	Anti-religious M (SD)	Pro-religious M (SD)	Extrinsic M (SD)	ANOVA Model 1		ANCOVA Model 2		ANCOVA Model 3		
Variable	n = 130	n = 58	n = 66	n = 47	F	*p*	F	*p*	F	*p*	eta^2
EAT total	8.65 (11.26)	12.06 (14.60)	13.31 (14.23)	16.15 (16.20)	5.84	0.001	12.34	0.001	11.69	0.001	0.06
EAT dieting	5.40 (6.91)	8.02 (9.06)	8.35 (9.14)	9.49 (9.78)	3.78	0.01	7.37	0.007	5.53	0.02	0.04
EAT bulimia	1.35 (3.06)	2.14 (4.33)	2.50 (3.84)	3.13 (4.32)	4.49	0.004	12.50	<0.001	13.38	<0.001	0.04
EAT Oral control	1.89 (3.18)	1.90 (3.61)	2.45 (3.62)	3.53 (4.14)	4.45	0.004	3.09	0.11	3.51	0.08	0.04
BSQ total	75.91 (28.10)	83.49 (35.9)	94.00 (34.21)	92.22 (34.96)	6.15	<0.001	29.85	<0.001	10.58	0.002	0.06

Note M mean, *SD* standard deviation, *EAT* Eating Attitudes Test, *BSQ* Body Shape Questionnaire. All analyses for the Eating Attitudes Test (EAT) and its subscales used logarithmically transformed values to correct for skewness. Non-transformed mean and standard deviation values are presented for ease of comparison. Variables used as covariates for model 2 were: age, body mass index (BMI), level of observance (orthodox Jewish vs. non-orthodox Jewish). Variables used as covariates for model 3 were: age, body mass index (BMI), level of observance, depressive symptoms, and trait anxiety. Data collection site was entered as a random effects variable for both ANCOVA models dependent variables. All ANOVAs were significant for religious orientation at or below the $p = 0.01$ level. Consistent with our hypothesis, an overall pattern of mean values existed for the intrinsic (lowest mean scores), anti-religious (next to lowest mean scores), pro-religious (next to highest mean scores), and extrinsic (highest mean scores) groups.

Post hoc comparisons for the total EAT score showed significant differences between the intrinsic and extrinsic groups ($p < 0.001$), intrinsic and pro-religious groups ($p = 0.01$), and the extrinsic and anti-religious groups ($p = 0.03$). For the EAT Dieting subscale, there were significant differences between the intrinsic and extrinsic groups ($p = 0.01$) and between the intrinsic and pro-religious groups ($p = 0.012$). For the EAT Bulimia subscale, there were significant differences between the intrinsic and extrinsic groups ($p = 0.001$), intrinsic and pro-religious groups ($p = 0.018$), and the extrinsic and anti-religious groups ($p = 0.046$). For the Eat Oral Control subscale, there were significant differences between the intrinsic and extrinsic groups ($p = 0.002$), the extrinsic and pro-religious groups ($p = 0.043$), and the extrinsic and anti- religious groups ($p = 0.001$). For the BSQ, there were significant differences between the intrinsic and extrinsic groups ($p = 0.01$), the intrinsic and pro-religious groups ($p < 0.001$), and the comparison between the pro-religious and anti-religious groups approached significance ($p = 0.07$). With the exception of the Oral Control subscale of the EAT, all results remained significant for both ANCOVA models. Data collection site was not significant in any of the models.

Spirituality and Eating Disorder Symptoms

Participants were categorized as being low, moderate, or high on each type of spiritual well-being. However, because the "low" groups had sample sizes of 2, 6, and 0 for the SWB, RWB and EWB respectively, they were eliminated and all analyses were conducted for those individuals categorized as either moderate or high on each type of well-being.

Spiritual Well-Being (SWB)

As shown in Table 13.2, for SWB, ANOVAs demonstrated significant differences only for the BSQ, $F(1,297) = 4.572$, $p = 0.033$, $d = 0.27$. Participants with moderate spiritual well-being had significantly higher scores on the BSQ than those with high spiritual well-being. This relationship remained significant when adjusting for demographic variables and for data collection site with ANCOVA in

Table 13.2 Influence of spiritual well-being on body dissatisfaction and eating disturbance

Spiritual well-being	Moderate M (SD)	High M (SD)	ANOVA Model 1		ANCOVA Model 2		ANCOVA Model 3		
Variable	n = 182	n = 117	F	*p*	F	*p*	F	*p*	*d*
EAT total	12.08 (14.08)	10.67 (13.14)	0.25	0.61	0.99	0.41	0.27	0.77	0.06
EAT dieting	7.46 (8.68)	6.8 (8.18)	0.08	0.78	1.13	0.37	0.48	0.63	0.03
EAT bulimia	2.18 (3.91)	1.8 (3.52)	0.28	0.60	0.53	0.53	0.15	0.86	0.06
EAT oral control	2.43 (3.69)	2.03 (3.36)	1.37	0.24	0.65	0.49	0.25	0.78	0.14
BSQ total	87.17 (34.40)	78.84 (30.36)	4.57	0.03	26.62	<0.001	0.37	0.69	0.26

Note M mean, *SD* standard deviation, *EAT* Eating Attitudes Test, *BSQ* Body Shape Questionnaire. All analyses for the Eating Attitudes Test (EAT) and its subscales used logarithmically transformed values to correct for skewness. Non-transformed mean and standard deviation values are presented for ease of comparison. Variables used as covariates for model 2 were: age, body mass index (BMI), and level of observance (orthodox Jewish vs. non-orthodox Jewish). Variables used as covariates for model 2 were: age, body mass index (BMI), level of observance, depressive symptoms, and trait anxiety. Data collection site was entered as a random effects variable for both ANCOVA models

model 2, but was no longer significant when also adjusting for mood variables with ANCOVA in model 3. Data collection site was not significant in any of the models.

Religious Well-Being

As shown in Table 13.3, there were no significant findings for RWB or any of the dependent variables.

Existential Well-Being (EWB)

As shown in Table 13.4, for EWB, ANOVAs showed significant differences only for the BSQ, $F(1,299) = 18.226$, $p < 0.001$, $d = 0.51$. Participants with moderate existential well-being had significantly higher scores on the BSQ than those with high existential well-being. This relationship remained significant when adjusting for demographic variables and data collection site with ANCOVA in model 2, but was no longer significant when also adjusting for mood variables with ANCOVA in model 3. Data collection site was not significant in any of the models.

Table 13.3 Influence of religious well-being on body dissatisfaction and eating disturbance

Religious well-being	Moderate M (SD)	High M (SD)	ANOVA Model 1		ANCOVA Model 2		ANCOVA Model 3		
Variable	n = 154	n = 141	F	*p*	F	*p*	F	*p*	*d*
EAT total	11.25 (12.67)	11.41 (14.45)	0.21	0.64	1.46	0.31	0.42	0.67	0.05
EAT dieting	6.99 (7.91)	7.14 (8.82)	0.01	0.91	0.82	0.39	0.47	0.63	0.01
EAT bulimia	1.90 (3.50)	2.04 (3.82)	0.01	0.92	0.23	0.66	0.12	0.89	0.01
EAT oral control	2.35 (3.46)	2.23 (3.72)	0.60	0.43	0.30	0.61	0.93	0.41	0.09
BSQ total	85.39 (33.31)	81.35 (31.86)	1.12	0.29	5.19	0.06	1.26	0.29	0.12

Note M mean, *SD* standard deviation, *EAT* Eating Attitudes Test, *BSQ* Body Shape Questionnaire. All analyses for the Eating Attitudes Test (EAT) and its subscales used logarithmically transformed values to correct for skewness. Non-transformed mean and standard deviation values are presented for ease of comparison. Variables used as covariates for model 2 were: age, body mass index (BMI), and level of observance (orthodox Jewish vs. non-orthodox Jewish). Variables used as covariates for model 3 were: age, body mass index (BMI), level of observance, depressive symptoms, and trait anxiety. Data collection site was entered as a random effects variable for both ANCOVA models

Table 13.4 Influence of existential well-being on body dissatisfaction and eating disturbance

Existential well-being	Moderate M (SD)	High M (SD)	ANOVA Model 1		ANCOVA Model 2		ANCOVA Model 3		
Variable	n = 179	n = 122	F	*p*	F	*p*	F	*p*	*d*
EAT total	12.62 (14.19)	9.84 (12.76)	2.61	0.11	1.41	0.35	0.08	0.81	0.19
EAT dieting	7.94 (8.90)	6.09 (7.67)	2.48	0.12	2.10	0.27	0.12	0.75	0.19
EAT bulimia	2.20 (3.88)	1.79 (3.56)	1.00	0.32	0.57	0.52	0.34	0.60	0.12
EAT oral control	2.48 (3.72)	1.97 (3.28)	2.26	0.13	1.41	0.35	0.60	0.50	0.17
BSQ total	90.56 (33.76)	74.47 (29.49)	18.23	<0.001	56.00	<0.001	1.67	0.20	0.51

Note M mean, *SD* standard deviation, *EAT* Eating Attitudes Test, *BSQ* Body Shape Questionnaire. All analyses for the Eating Attitudes Test (EAT) and its subscales used logarithmically transformed values to correct for skewness. Non-transformed mean and standard deviation values are presented for ease of comparison. Variables used as covariates for model 2 were: age, body mass index (BMI), and level of observance (orthodox Jewish vs. non-orthodox Jewish). Variables used as covariates for model 3 were: age, body mass index (BMI), level of observance depressive symptoms, and trait anxiety. Data collection site was entered as a random effects variable for both ANCOVA models

Discussion

Study results confirmed our hypotheses and revealed that religious orientation is strongly associated with body dissatisfaction and eating disturbance. Participants with an intrinsic religious orientation had consistently lower scores (indicating less pathology) on measures of body dissatisfaction and eating disturbance than participants with an extrinsic, pro-religious, or anti-religious orientation. Also, there was a moderate association between spiritual well-being and body dissatisfaction and eating disturbance.

Religious Orientation and ED Symptoms

We measured religious orientation using the religious orientation scale (ROS), which distinguishes between intrinsic and extrinsic religious orientations. Intrinsically oriented individuals tend to internalize and live their religious beliefs, while extrinsically oriented individuals tend to engage in religious activities because of the social rewards or motivators associated with these activities. Individuals classified as pro-religious endorse intrinsic and extrinsic items, and those classified as anti-religious tend to disagree with items from both domains. We assessed spirituality using the spiritual well-being scale (SWB), which distinguishes between different types of spirituality as being related to or distinct from religious practice. Consistent with our first hypothesis, participants categorized as having an intrinsic religious orientation as measured by the ROS, had lower scores on both the EAT (and its subscales) and the BSQ than participants categorized as extrinsic, pro-religious, and anti-religious. These findings remained significant after controlling for age, BMI, observance level, depression, anxiety and data collection site—and were consistent with results from previous studies, which did not include Jewish women [18, 19].

According to study results, it appears that internalizing one's religious beliefs is helpful in terms of the development of body image and eating disturbance as compared to having an extrinsic attitude. Extrinsically oriented individuals often focus on the social or external rewards that religious practice can provide and may be more outwardly focused on physical appearance. It is noteworthy that with the exception of the Oral Control subscale of the EAT, the extrinsic and pro-religious groups did not differ significantly from each other. Participants categorized as pro-religious endorsed both intrinsic and extrinsic items and scored similarly to those with an extrinsic orientation, suggesting that the deleterious effects of an extrinsic orientation may outweigh the protective effects of an intrinsic one. Interestingly, while the intrinsic group had the lowest scores on all EAT subscales and the BSQ, this group was often not significantly different from the anti-religious group, whose members tended to disagree with both intrinsic and extrinsic items. This suggests that perhaps as long as one does not actually endorse and extrinsic orientation, this too may be protective against body image and eating disturbance.

Studies of Jewish women that have found that an increased level of observance or orthodoxy is associated with lower levels of body dissatisfaction and eating disorders, have attributed religion's emphasis on the spiritual (as opposed to the physical) as the basis for this difference [13, 14]. Gluck and Geliebter [13] asserted that among Orthodox Jewish women, there is little emphasis on being thin and being successful outside the home, which may confer protection against body dissatisfaction. Furthermore, they argued that the rigidity of an orthodox lifestyle, which includes observing the Sabbath and dietary laws of Kashrut [9], may provide a feeling of control for its constituents, eliminating the need to use the body as a vehicle of control. While this may be true to some extent, it is likely an oversimplification of the values of orthodox Judaism. Among this population, exploration of religious orientation rather than observance appears to enhance understanding of the role that religion plays in ED development.

An issue not considered in previous empirical studies of orthodox Jewish women and body image is the extreme pressure within this community to enter into a socially desirable marriage at an early age [10, 11, 29, 30]. Even among segments of this population with limited exposure to media, ideas about what constitutes a "suitable" bride closely resemble unattainable beauty ideals portrayed in the mainstream media. In fact, some have observed that over the last decade, the acceptable weight for orthodox women of marriageable age has become thinner and thinner, while beauty ideals have become more rigid [10, 11]. Orthodox Jewish women not only are expected to conform to rigid appearance standards, but they also are expected to do so within the boundaries of Tzniut or modesty laws. Briefly, these laws prohibit women and girls over 12 years of age from exposing any skin above the elbows or knees as well as the chest area below the collarbone [31], and many women also cover the lower legs with stockings. While the essence of these laws is about modesty and self-respect, they often are rigidly enforced and may be misinterpreted by adolescent and young women. For example, they may serve to induce shame about one's body or sexuality. Furthermore, for many Orthodox girls, formal dating for marriage is the first real interaction with boys, and all physical and sexual contact is prohibited until after marriage [9]. Contrary to Gluck and Geliebter's assertion that this rigid lifestyle provides a sense of control, many young women have reported feeling extremely "out of control" as a result of orthodox Jewish tenets; these women may use their bodies in unhealthy ways (e.g., food restriction or bingeing) as a way to express uncomfortable or shameful feelings [10, 29].

In the context of the values and standards reported above, orthodox Jewish women may feel even more pressure than their secular counterparts to conform to a thin-ideal. This is where the distinction between an intrinsic and extrinsic orientation becomes crucial and is more useful than the simple distinction between observant versus non-observant or orthodox versus non-orthodox. As suggested by our findings, participants with an extrinsic orientation towards religion, who are concerned primarily with its social aspects, may be more outwardly focused on physical appearance, especially as it relates to community pressures. By contrast, intrinsically oriented individuals may be better able to distinguish societal pressures from religious values. These women may in fact be the ones who are protected by Orthodox Judaism's values, whereas women with an extrinsic orientation may be more vulnerable to body dissatisfaction and eating disturbance. In this regard, religious orientation is a more appropriate paradigm for measuring religious attitudes among secular and observant women alike. It is possible that the element of increased religiosity that appears protective in previous studies is actually intrinsic religiosity, as observed in the current study, rather than mere observance. With regard to Latzer et al. [14], it is possible that religiosity (or observance level) within Israeli society is more closely related to the idea of religious orientation than it is in the United States. While ED rates in Israel are comparable to those in the United States, cultural pressures within the orthodox community in Israel may be different than those in the United States. An expansion of the paradigm of religious orientation to Israeli women may or may not yield a similar pattern of results. Replicating the current study within other Jewish communities and among clinical samples is necessary to fully understand the association between religious orientation and ED symptoms among Jewish women.

Spiritual Well-Being and ED Symptoms

An important study goal was to examine the influence of spirituality on eating disturbance as a distinct construct from religion. Spirituality may or may not be related to religious practice, as many individuals report being spiritual but not religious and vice versa [16]. The majority of research related to religion and health has used the terms "religion" and "spirituality" interchangeably and has failed to address the possibility that, as separate constructs, they may have differing degrees of influence on health outcomes including body image and eating disturbance. The spiritual well-being scale (SWB), which was used to measure spirituality in the current study, includes the subscales of religious and existential well-being (RWB and EWB). Religious well-being refers specifically to one's relationship with God and religious practice, whereas existential well-being refers to welfare independent of God or religion, and includes feelings of fulfillment and purpose in life. The two subscales can be combined to obtain a total SWB score.

Our results indicated that for the BSQ, participants who scored high on total SWB and EWB had significantly lower scores than those with moderate SWB and EWB, suggesting that higher levels of spiritual well-being may be protective against body dissatisfaction. These findings remained significant when controlling for demographic variables but were no longer significant after controlling for mood variables. There were no differences on the EAT or its subscales and no differences on any measure for RWB.

These findings highlight several important issues. First, a possible explanation for the finding of group differences on the BSQ but not the EAT, relates to the fact that the BSQ measures overall body dissatisfaction whereas the EAT measures actual disordered eating. It is likely that many of our participants exhibited body dissatisfaction without having progressed to disordered eating behaviors. One might consider the BSQ a more cognitive measure of risk factors for EDs because it measures thoughts and self-perceptions, which likely become distorted prior to the development of disordered eating behaviors [32]. As such, individuals are likely to have elevated scores on measures of body dissatisfaction prior to having elevated scores on measures of eating disturbance. Therefore, in our non-clinical sample, one might expect to find greater variation in scores on the BSQ than on the EAT.

Second, statistically significant outcomes on measures of body dissatisfaction between those with moderate and high SWB and EWB disappeared after controlling for depression and anxiety. This is likely due to the nature of the spiritual well-being scale. Because the scale measures spiritual well-being, and not spirituality per se, it is likely that scores were related to mood variables such as anxiety and depression. Because individuals with high scores on measures of body dissatisfaction are also likely to have high scores on tests of anxiety and depression [3, 32], group differences may disappear after controlling for these variables. Overall, these findings suggest that the spiritual well-being scale may not be the most useful measure of spirituality when conducting psychological research or when utilizing participant groups in which psychopathology might be present, even at subclinical levels.

Lastly, there was no observed influence of RWB. One could argue that RWB, as assessed via the Spiritual Well-Being scale, is not a true measure of spirituality but rather a measure of how one perceives his or her relationship with God. When arguing that spirituality should be considered as distinct from religion, it follows that EWB is of greater interest than RWB because RWB may be more related to religiosity or observance than to spirituality. If this were the case, then one would expect RWB to be of little value in predicting eating disturbance, given our other findings (described above), which highlighted the limitations of using observance alone as a predictor of disordered eating. Thus, it makes sense that these results revealed significant differences only for total SWB and EWB—and researchers should bear in mind this potential limitation when designing future studies dealing with spirituality.

Study Limitations and Future Directions

Several study limitations warrant mention. As discussed above, the utility of the spiritual well-being scale may be limited. When looking at the influence of SWB on body dissatisfaction and eating disturbance, significant results disappeared after controlling for depression and anxiety, suggesting that the scale is measuring a construct closely related to these mood variables. Because it appears that the subscale of EWB most closely resembles the construct of spirituality as being distinct from religious practice, a possible option is to utilize this subscale exclusively in future studies. In order to understand fully whether spirituality (as a separate construct from religion) influences ED symptomatology, additional spirituality measures should be utilized and/or developed.

The current study did not inquire about participants' marital status, which will be included in future studies. Given the emphasis placed on marrying at a young age within the orthodox community and the demands associated with it, a comparison of married versus non-married participants might yield important findings. It may be useful to include measures of personality, such as extraversion and neuroticism. Because these personality variables are associated with a variety of health outcomes [33], they may inform and/or impact both religious orientation and attitudes towards one's body.

Another future goal is to examine whether the paradigm of religious orientation extends to other religious and cultural groups as well as to other Jewish communities such as those in Israel. Results of this study are similar to those seen in previous research with a predominantly Christian sample [8]. If studies conducted among different religious groups and denominations continue to show that having an intrinsic orientation acts as a buffer for the development of ED symptoms, then religious orientation may emerge as an effective tool for measuring the influence of religion in ED development. Additionally, studies using religious orientation should be expanded to include boys and young men, whose rates of body image and eating disturbance have been steadily increasing [34]. Thus, religious orientation can be added to the general repertoire of research tools available to elucidate the etiology of EDs.

Study Implications

The rationale underlying the quest for a deeper understanding of ED development is to enable the successful design and implementation of interventions aimed at vulnerable populations. While members of the orthodox Jewish community may be resistant to discussing matters related to psychiatric illness [10, 29], it is nevertheless imperative to disseminate information that has the potential to protect young women from developing EDs. Over the last several years, some Yeshivas and Jewish day schools have begun to provide workshops and seminars aimed at prevention and early detection of eating disturbance [29], and incorporating information related to intrinsic and extrinsic orientations would add to these efforts. As well, parents and school administrations should be encouraged to engage in open dialogue about the messages that are being transmitted to young women regarding what determines self-worth. Arguably, the importance of marriage and children, which are at the core of Jewish values, can be emphasized in a way that does not detract from women's inherent value. Furthermore, community and educational efforts may be initiated to expand the image of what constitutes a "suitable bride." This could involve educational programs aimed at young women and men that reinforce healthy and realistic beauty standards. Ideally, school counselors and psychologists (who are knowledgeable about these and related study findings) would be involved in all of the endeavors described above.

Study findings also may be used to inform treatment. For example, an awareness of different religious orientations and their implications would be beneficial to clinicians working with patients who manifest eating disorders and body image disturbances. It may even be possible to design therapeutic and/or experimental interventions that challenge existing attitudes and encourage an intrinsic religious orientation. If successful, such efforts might exert a positive effect not only on body image and eating disturbance but on other mental health outcomes as well.

Conclusions

Merely using self-reported attendance at religious services or observance level is of little use in evaluating religion's connection with health. Without a sophisticated understanding of how individuals incorporate religious beliefs into their lives and what motivates them to do so, religion's true impact on real-world outcomes may be overlooked. It is hoped that the current study can serve as a starting point for such efforts. This study showed that having an intrinsic religious orientation is related to lower scores on measures of body dissatisfaction and eating disturbance and may confer protection from the internalization of unhealthy media ideals. It is reasonable to assume that the influences of religious orientation may extend to other mental and physical health outcomes. Using religious orientation as a means of understanding individuals' true religious attitudes can provide a mechanism by which to gain a more comprehensive understanding of how religion affects a variety of mental and physical health outcomes, including depression, happiness, coping, and recovery from illness.

Take home points

- Intrinsic religious orientation (the manner in which people are connected to their religious attitudes and faiths) is related to reduced body dissatisfaction and eating disturbance to a greater extent than extrinsic religious orientation (belonging to a religious community).
- Intrinsic religious orientation may protect from the internalization of unhealthy media ideals.
- It is reasonable to assume that the influences of religious orientation may extend to other mental and physical health domains in addition to EDs.
- Using religious orientation as a means of understanding the individuals' religious attitudes can assist in gaining a more comprehensive understanding of how religion may affect a variety of mental and physical health-related outcomes, including coping with illness and recovery from it.

Acknowledgments This study was derived from the first author's doctoral dissertation, conducted at Brooklyn College and the Graduate Center of the City University of New York. Dr. Weinberger-Litman is currently a postdoctoral research fellow at the Mount Sinai School of Medicine.

References

1. Brumberg JJ. Fasting girls: The history of anorexia nervosa. New York: Vintage Books; 2000.
2. Keel P, Klump KL. Are eating disorders culture-bound syndromes? Implications for conceptualizing their etiology. Psychol Bull. 2003;129:747–69.
3. Walsh BT, Devlin MJ. Eating disorders: Progress and problems. Science. 1998;280:1387–90.
4. Vince EM, Walker I. A set of meta-analytic studies on the factors associated with disordered eating. Internet J Ment Health. 2008, in press.
5. Vandereycken W, Van Deth R. From fasting saints to anorexic girls. New York: University Press; 1994.
6. Lelwica MM. Starving for Salvation. New York: Oxford Univ Press; 1999.
7. Joughin N, Crisp AH, Halek C, Humphrey H. Religious belief and anorexia nervosa. Int J Eat Disord. 1992;12:397–406.
8. Smith FT, Hardman RK, Richards PS, Fischer L. Intrinsic religiousness and spiritual well-being as predictors of treatment outcome among women with eating disorders. Eat Disord. 2003;11:15–26.
9. Ganzfried S. Code of Jewish law. Goldin HE, Trans. New York: Hebrew Publ Co, 1961. (Original work published 1864).
10. Altmann E. Eating disorders in the Jewish community. MyJewishLearning.com. Accessed August 22, 2007, from http://www.myjewishlearning.com/daily_life/TheBody/Health_Healing/Caring_for_Ones_Health/eatingdisorders.htm.
11. Dancyger I, Fornari V, Fisher M. Cultural factors in Orthodox Jewish adolescents treated in a day program for eating disorders. Int J Adolesc Med Health. 2002;14:317–28.
12. Kim KH. Religion, weight perception, and weight control behavior. Eat Behav. 2007;8: 121–31.
13. Gluck ME, Geliebter A. Body image and eating behaviors in Orthodox and secular Jewish women. J Gend Specif Med. 2002;5:19–24.
14. LatzerY, Tzischinsky O, Gefen S. Level of religiosity and disordered eating related behaviors among Orthodox Jewish adolescents in Israel. Int J Adolesc Med Health. 2007;19:511–21.
15. Powell LH, Shahabi L, Thoreson CE. Religion and spirituality: Linkages to physical health. Am Psychol. 2003;58:36–52.
16. Miller WR, Thoresen CE. Spirituality, religion and health: An emerging research field. Am Psychol. 2003;58:24–35.
17. Allport GW, Ross JM. Personal religious orientation and prejudice. J Pers Soc Psychol. 1967;5:432–43.
18. Smith MH, Richards PS, Maglio CJ. Examining the relationship between religious orientation and eating disturbances. Eat Behav. 2004;5:171–80.
19. Forthun LF, Pidcock BW, Fischer JL. Religiousness and disordered eating: Does religiousness modify family risk? Eat Behav. 2003;4:7–26.
20. Garner DM, Garfinkel PM. The eating attitudes test: An index of symptoms in anorexia nervosa. Psychol Med. 1979;9:273–9.
21. Garner DM, Olmstead MP, Bohr Y, Garfinkel PM. The Eating Attitudes Test: Psychometric features and clinical correlates. Psychol Med. 1982;12:871–8.
22. Cooper PJ, Taylor MJ, Cooper Z, Fairburn CG. The development of the body shape questionnaire. Int J E Disord. 1987;6:485–94.
23. Donahue MJ. Intrinsic and extrinsic religiousness: Review and meta analysis. J Pers Soc Psychol. 1985;48:400–19.
24. Paloutzian RE, Ellison CW. Manual for the spiritual well-being scale. Nyack, NY: Life Advance; 1991.
25. Ellison CW, Smith J. Toward an integrative measure of health and well-being. J Psychol Theol. 1991;19:35–8.
26. Beck AT, Steer RA, Garbin MG. Psychometric properties of the Beck Depression Inventory: Twenty-five years of evaluation. Clin Psychol Rev. 1988;8:77–100.

27. Spielberger CD, Edwards CD, Lushene RE, Montuori J, Platzek D. Preliminary manual for the state-trait anxiety inventory for children. Palo Alto, CA: Consult Psychol Press; 1973.
28. Becker LE. Online effect size calculator 1999. Revised October, 2004. Accessed March 1, 2007, from http://web.uccs.edu/lbecker/Psy590/escalc3.htm.
29. Baruchin A. What can Orthodox girls control? Lilith. 1998;23:8.
30. Goldwasser D. Starving to live. New York: Judaica Press; 2000.
31. Falk PE. Modesty: An adornment for life. Nanuet, New York: Feldheim; 1998.
32. Keel PK, Baxter MG, Heatherton TF, Joiner TE Jr. A 20-year longitudinal study of body weight, dieting, and eating disorder symptoms. J Abnorm Psychol. 2007;116:422–32.
33. Taylor SE. Health Psychology. New York: McGraw-Hill; 2005.
34. Hudson JI, Hiripi E, Pope HG Jr, Kessler RC. The prevalence and correlates of eating disorders in the national comorbidity survey replication. Biol Psychiatry. 2007;61:348–5.

MIX
Papier aus verantwortungsvollen Quellen
Paper from responsible sources
FSC® C105338

If you have any concerns about our products,
you can contact us on
ProductSafety@springernature.com

In case Publisher is established outside the EU,
the EU authorized representative is:
Springer Nature Customer Service Center GmbH
Europaplatz 3, 69115 Heidelberg, Germany

Printed by Libri Plureos GmbH
in Hamburg, Germany